LOSE WEIGHT
WITH YOUR
INSTANT POT

ALSO BY AUDREY JOHNS

Lose Weight by Eating:
130 Amazing Clean-Eating Recipe Makeovers
for Guilt-Free Comfort Food

Lose Weight by Eating: Detox Week

LOSE WEIGHT
WITH YOUR
INSTANT POT

60 Easy One-Pot Recipes for Fast Weight Loss

Audrey Johns

wm

WILLIAM MORROW

An Imprint of HarperCollins*Publishers*

FIRST EDITION

Designed by Suet Yee Chong
Photography by Carl Kravats

Library of Congress Cataloging-in-Publication Data has been applied for.

ISBN 978-0-06-287455-9

18 19 20 21 22 ID/LSC 10 9 8 7 6 5 4 3 2 1

For Kate, the woman who taught me to cook.
I would not be a cookbook author without you.
You were a dear friend, an inspiration,
and always a bright spot in my life.

To Ruby and Violet, I love you, sweet girls.
Know that your beautiful mama was an amazing woman,
she loved you very much, and she will always be with you.

You will be missed, my dear.
This book is for you.

CONTENTS

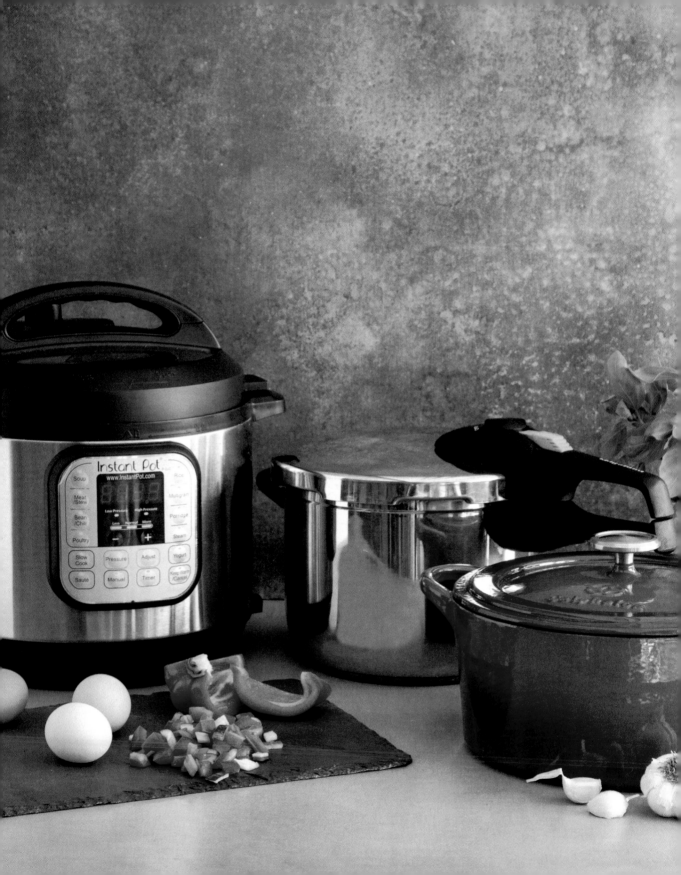

Introduction

One cold Monday night I got a text message from my literary agent, Sarah, saying, "Hi!! Give me a call when you have a moment!!" I was at drum class with my daughter, Sophia, and I ducked outside into the winter chill to call her. My second cookbook had just come out, so I assumed it was about that book.

"We have an idea," she said. "Do you want to write an Instant Pot cookbook?" I was excited to write a book showcasing my healthy comfort food in the popular electronic pressure cooker—it seemed like a match made in heaven! Within a week I had my Instant Pot out and was testing recipes.

Instant Pots have been featured on many online cooking boards, where people often say, "I've had my IP for six months and finally took it out of the box today—why did I wait so long?" That's how many feel about this equipment . . . it's a little daunting to use the first time, but once you get started, you're hooked!

A month later I had two different sizes of Instant Pot, a 6-quart and a 3-quart (or Momma Bear and Baby Bear, as I named them). Soon I was using them daily! They defy all the "rules" I know about cooking . . . such as that brownies need to be baked (see page 131 for my IP brownie recipe), or a good marinara sauce needs to cook for at least four hours (see page 63 for my thirty-minute IP recipe). I was able to make dinner and walk away for three hours (leaving it on warm) to come home to the best sloppy joes (page 31) I've ever had.

So if you haven't yet embraced the Instant Pot, open the box and get started—it's easier than it seems! And if you already love your IP, enjoy these skinny recipes to help you slim down and enjoy the comfort food you know and love.

Happy cooking,
XO Audrey

1

INSTANT POT BASICS

What's so special about the Instant Pot?

Some of you will be new to the Instant Pot and others will already be well versed in the equipment. Here's why I love this amazing piece of kitchen gear:

- I can cook a meal in a fraction of the time. I have a busy life, and often I realize late in the afternoon that I have nothing planned for dinner. Instant Pot meals can be finished in a matter of moments. I can walk away from the pot to get ready in the morning while it cooks my breakfast, or to do homework with my kiddo in the afternoon and trust that dinner will come out perfectly without any effort on my part.

- I love the "keep warm" feature on the Instant Pot. Recently I made Chicken Tortilla Soup (page 52) and was able to leave the house to attend a Girl Scout troop meeting and come home to dinner. Just as with the slow cooker, you can walk away and come back to a perfect meal, and that makes it great for my busy schedule.

- I can make almost anything in the Instant Pot! From breakfast to dessert and everything in between—it's a lifesaver!

- I love how easy the cleanup is, since you can make a whole meal in one pot (or two if I need both of my Instant Pots . . . yes, I have two). Not a sauté pan, a pot, and a casserole dish.

- I love that my kiddo can help out. There's no open flame, so it's a great device for teaching a child to cook! She loves to add all the ingredients and press the buttons. And kids are always more open to trying new things when they have helped prepare them.

Key Instructions and Tips

Just a bit of housekeeping before we get started, to help you make the recipes in this book. I'll keep this short and sweet, as most of this will be in your Instant Pot manual.

There are lots of fun buttons on your Instant Pot, but each model is a little bit different (for instance, my Instant Pots don't have a "yogurt" button). So I tried to stick to the settings that are universal: "sauté," "egg," "manual," and "keep warm/cancel."

HIGH PRESSURE

When a recipe instructs you to cook on high pressure, that simply means you cover the pot, close the valve, and hit the "manual" button.

LIGHTLY COVERED

A couple of the recipes say to lightly cover your pot. Some Instant Pots come with a glass lid, and you can use that here, or you can use the regular Instant Pot lid. But if you do, set the lid a bit askew so that it's covering the pot but not settled into the machine.

QUICK RELEASE

When you're instructed to do a quick release, use a wooden spoon to push the pressure valve to "venting." Be sure to approach it from the side—not from above—to avoid burning yourself. The steam that comes out of the pressure valve is extremely hot, so use the wooden spoon for safety.

NATURAL RELEASE

When directed to do a natural release, just let the Instant Pot sit until the pressure releases on its own.

SAUTÉ

The "sauté" setting is just like cooking on a stovetop, and you can always use a pan on the stovetop instead, though it will create more dirty dishes. Be sure to watch and stir what you're cooking on the sauté setting, as it can burn.

FOIL SLING

Some recipes call for you to make a foil sling, which will help you lift items out of the pot without burning yourself. (You can also buy one as an Instant Pot accessory, but it's easy to do with your household foil.) Here's how you do it:

STEP 1: Pull off a 3-foot-long piece of foil.
STEP 2: Fold the foil in half crosswise to make a 1½-foot-long piece of foil.
STEP 3: On the side with the cut edges, fold in a 2-inch-wide piece, then keep folding it over and over again, until you have a thick, 2-inch-wide strip of foil.

To use your foil sling, set it in the pot before you place the items or use it to lower large baking dishes into the pot (such as the 7-inch round baking dish in the Prosciutto and Asparagus Strata, page 12) that may need lifting. When you use the Instant Pot, be sure the foil is tucked all the way inside the pot so that the pot can seal well.

I know this may seem like an awful lot of foil, but you need the sling to be strong enough to lift heavy dishes out of the Instant Pot. I use my sling over and over again until it's charred, so it's not a huge waste of foil.

STEAMER BASKET

There are lots of fancy gadgets you can purchase for your Instant Pot, but I tried to limit the special equipment called for in this book. A few recipes, such as the Protein Bowl (page 33), do call for a steamer basket, which is inexpensive and very handy—you can even use it in a stovetop pot!

I wanted to mention the basket here, as it does not come with your Instant Pot. I picked mine up at my local grocery store, but you can also find them online for about $5.

Weight Loss with Your Instant Pot

In this book and my two others, *Lose Weight by Eating* and *Lose Weight by Eating: Detox Week*, I've taken my favorite comfort food recipes and made them healthier and all natural, packing them full of metabolism-boosting ingredients to help the food do the weight-loss work for you. Weight loss is found in the kitchen, not in a gym and not in a magic pill.

For years now I've worked with people who can't exercise, some due to an injury or disability and others due to time and basic life constraints. I myself lost 150 pounds in eleven months without exercising at all (due to an injury). I've kept it off for eight years, and just recently found a new love for exercise. Now, I'm not saying that exercise isn't helpful or good for you. It is! I like to tell people weight loss comes from the kitchen, but a lean, fit body comes from a gym (or other fitness plan). Can you lose weight without exercising? *Yes!* Can you have a firm, fit body without exercise? Sadly, no.

With that said, think of me as your kitchen trainer, sharing my tips and tricks to trim down with food. See your personal trainer to build muscle, increase cardio health, tone up after weight loss, and for overall health—and see me for recipes that will help you lose weight fast.

For this book, I took some of the most popular Instant Pot recipes and trimmed hundreds of calories from them (such as the Skinny "Crack" Chicken on page 49). I also created Instant Pot recipes that can raise your metabolism, suppress your appetite, and help you drop weight fast. I've included nutrition information, so if you have a diet plan you already love, you can incorporate these recipes into it.

While you're on your weight-loss journey, be sure to drink lots of water and stay within serving sizes. If you're looking for more weight-loss assistance, check out my other cookbooks for weight-loss plans that work with all of these recipes. You can also visit my website, www.loseweightbyeating.com, for weight-loss plans and assistance.

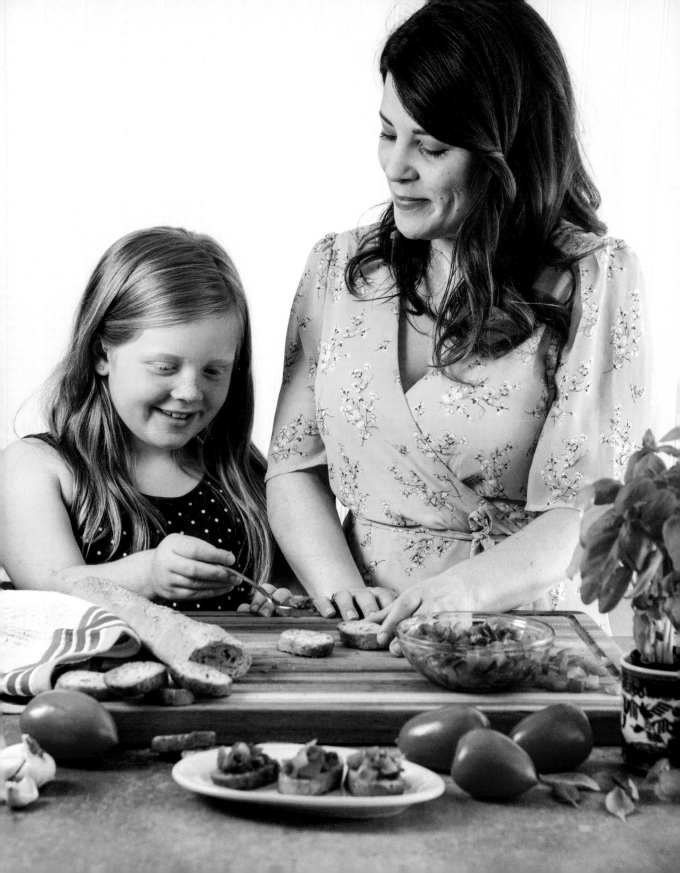

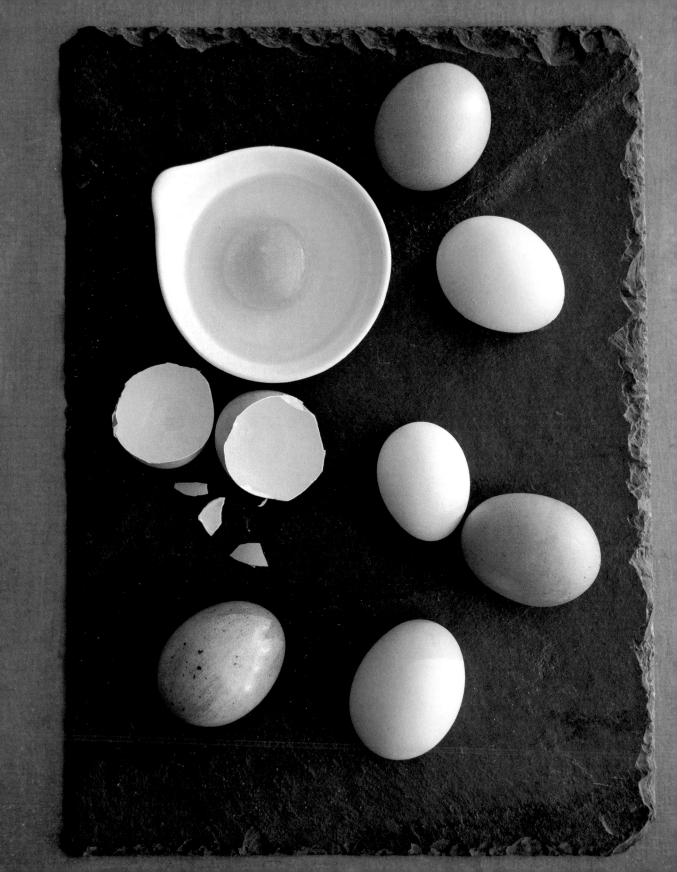

2

BREAKFASTS

One of the reasons I love my Instant Pot so much is that I can walk away from it while it cooks my meal. This gives me time to do important things, like take a shower or get my daughter ready for school.

If you find yourself too busy to cook in the mornings, try some of these dishes. The Orange-Cranberry Oatmeal (page 10) is fantastic and an easy "mix and walk away" kind of meal. The Homemade Yogurt with Fruit Topping Bar (page 19) can be made ahead for even more hectic mornings. And the Shakshuka (page 21) is so elegant, it will impress your brunch guests in a flash.

Orange-Cranberry Oatmeal

This hearty and flavorful oatmeal is anything but mushy and bland! I love incorporating citrus zest in my morning bowl; it adds a burst of flavor without any calories. This recipe would also taste great with lemon zest instead of orange zest, and you can swap your favorite unsweetened dried fruit for the cranberries. Versatile and delicious!

Makes 2 servings | Serving size: ¾ cup | Cook time: 35 minutes | Prep time: 3 minutes
Per serving: calories 97; fat 3.5 g; saturated fat 0.5 g; fiber 4 g; protein 5 g;
carbohydrates 21 g; sugar 5 g

½ cup steel-cut oats

Grated zest of ½ orange

Juice of 1 orange

2 tablespoons dried cranberries

1½ cups water

2 teaspoons chopped pecans

2 teaspoons pure maple syrup (optional)

1. In the Instant Pot, combine the oats, orange zest, orange juice, cranberries, and water. Cover and cook on high pressure for 10 minutes. Let the pressure release naturally for 10 minutes, then quick-release the remaining pressure.

2. If the oats are still watery, let sit uncovered for 5 minutes. The oatmeal will absorb the water.

3. Top with the pecans and maple syrup (if using).

Avocado Eggs

Avocados are packed full of potassium and healthy fats that actually tell your body to release fat. Yep, eat healthy fats and you will lose fat!

This filling meal is great alone, but if you need a heartier meal, add a slice of whole-grain toast to your plate and get some healthy, filling carbs with your protein-packed avocado egg.

Makes 2 servings │ Serving size: ½ avocado │ Cook time: 5 minutes │ Prep time: 3 minutes
Per serving: calories 315; fat 25 g; saturated fat 5.5 g; fiber 7 g; protein 13 g;
carbohydrates 11 g; sugar 2 g

---

1 avocado

2 large eggs

2 tablespoons grated sharp cheddar cheese

Kosher salt and freshly ground black pepper

1 cup water

1 tablespoon chopped fresh cilantro (optional)

Hot sauce or salsa (optional)

1. Halve the avocado and remove the pit. Use a spoon to scoop out one-quarter of the avocado flesh to make the hole in the center large enough to hold the egg. (I enjoy the excess avocado as a chef's treat . . . snacking while cooking is so satisfying.)

2. Crack an egg into each avocado well. Top each avocado egg with a sprinkling of cheese, and salt and pepper to taste.

3. Pour the water into the Instant Pot and set the rack inside. Gently set the avocado halves on the rack. Cover, choose the "egg" setting, and cook for 2 minutes.

4. For runny yolks, quick-release the pressure. For firm yolks, let the pressure release naturally for 5 minutes, then quick-release the remaining pressure.

5. Move each avocado half to a plate and top with cilantro and your favorite hot sauce or salsa, if desired.

Prosciutto and Asparagus Strata

You may notice that there are some ingredients I use several times in this book, and prosciutto is one of them. I do this for a few reasons: First, it helps to cut down on your grocery bill; second, it cuts down on food waste; and finally . . . if there is prosciutto in the house, *I will eat it!* So I need to find ways to use it in recipes, or I will gobble it up.

If you're like me and it isn't safe to have extra prosciutto in your house, turn to page 75 for another yummy recipe using this fantastic ingredient.

Makes 6 servings | Serving size: about ¾ cup | Cook time: 35 minutes | Prep time: 10 minutes
Per serving: calories 110; fat 7 g; saturated fat 2.5 g; fiber 2 g; protein 7 g;
carbohydrates 6 g; sugar 4 g

---

5 slices whole wheat bread (I save and
    freeze the heels just for this recipe)
Olive oil spray
3 thin slices prosciutto
½ red onion, cut into medium dice
3 large eggs
1 cup almond milk (or fat-free dairy milk)
Kosher salt and freshly ground black
    pepper
1½ cups water
1-pound bunch asparagus, trimmed and
    cut into 1-inch bites
4 tablespoons shredded sharp cheddar
    cheese

1. Cut the bread into ½-inch cubes, place on a rimmed baking sheet, and leave it out overnight to get stale. (Alternatively, toast the bread, then cube it.)

2. Line a plate with paper towels. Lightly coat a 12-inch skillet with olive oil spray and set it over medium-low heat. Add the prosciutto and cook for 3 to 5 minutes on each side, until crispy. Transfer to the prepared plate to drain. Add the onion to the skillet and sauté for 3 minutes, until just starting to soften.

3. Coat a 7-inch round baking dish with olive oil spray and make a foil sling (see page 5).

4. In a large bowl, whisk together the eggs and milk. Add a pinch each of salt and pepper and the bread cubes and mix to coat. Let sit for 5 minutes.

5. While the bread sits, pour the water into the Instant Pot and set the rack inside.

6. Add the onion, asparagus, and 2 tablespoons of the cheese to the bread, mix well, and spread in the prepared baking dish. Sprinkle the remaining cheese over the top and use the foil sling to lower the dish into the pot. Leave the sling in and cover the pot.

7. Cover and cook on high pressure for 15 minutes. Quick-release the pressure. Carefully lift the dish out of the pot with the help of the sling. It will be hot—wear oven mitts!

8. Use a large spoon to scoop out 6 servings and enjoy.

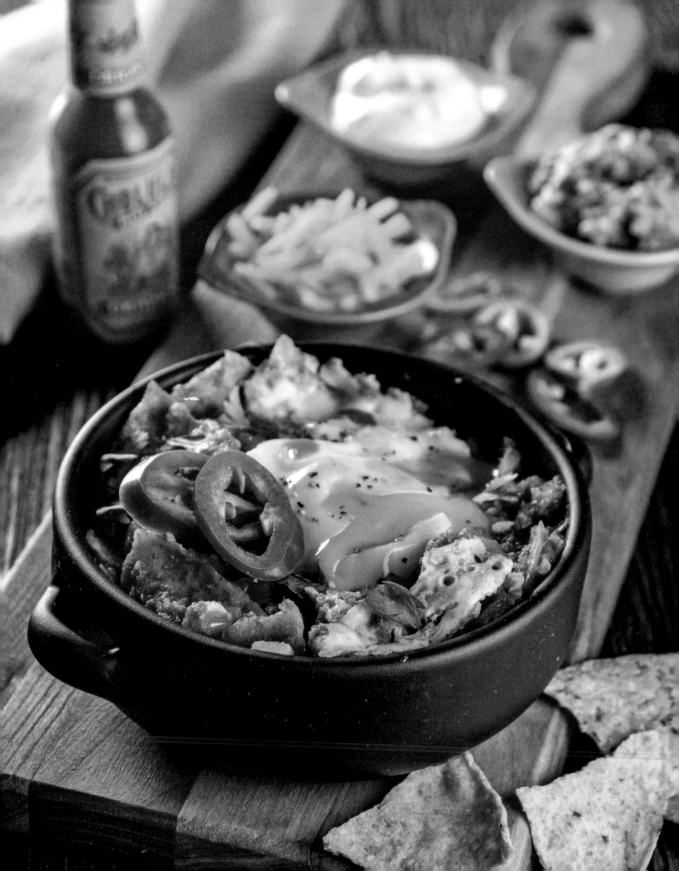

Chilaquiles

Oh, man . . . tortilla chips and eggs. Need I say more?! This is the perfect brunch meal . . . and by brunch, I mean hangover. You don't have to be hungover to enjoy this, but if you are, this is the cure-all! Be sure to add lots of your favorite hot sauce to burn off the booze and help revive you, and while you're cooking, start drinking water. That is what you really need . . . well, water and chilaquiles (wink).

One note: If you have stale tortilla chips, use them here! They'll get soft in the sauce anyhow.

Makes 3 servings │ Serving size: 1 egg and ⅓ cup chips │ Cook time: 15 minutes │
Prep time: 8 minutes
Per serving: calories 468; fat 11 g; saturated fat 2.5 g; fiber 13 g; protein 14 g;
carbohydrates 83 g; sugar 8 g

---

5 Roma (plum) tomatoes, cut into
    large chunks
2 jalapeños, seeds and ribs removed
1 teaspoon olive oil
½ red onion, roughly chopped
3 garlic cloves, minced
20 corn tortilla chips
3 large eggs
Kosher salt and freshly ground black
    pepper

OPTIONAL TOPPINGS
1 avocado, sliced
Chopped fresh cilantro
Greek yogurt (tastes just like sour cream)
Grated sharp cheddar cheese
Hot sauce

1. In a blender, combine the tomatoes and jalapeños and blend until smooth.

2. Set the Instant Pot to "sauté, medium heat." Once it reads "hot," add the olive oil and onion and sauté until veggies start to soften, about 5 minutes, stirring to avoid burning. Add the garlic and sauté for 2 minutes, then add the tomato mixture and sauté until bubbling, about 3 minutes. Hit "cancel."

3. Add the chips and stir to coat with the tomato sauce. Make 3 wells in the tortilla chips and crack the eggs into the wells. Sprinkle lightly with salt and pepper.

4. Cover and cook on high pressure for 1 minute. Quick-release the pressure. Scoop out the servings to 3 plates. Add toppings, if desired.

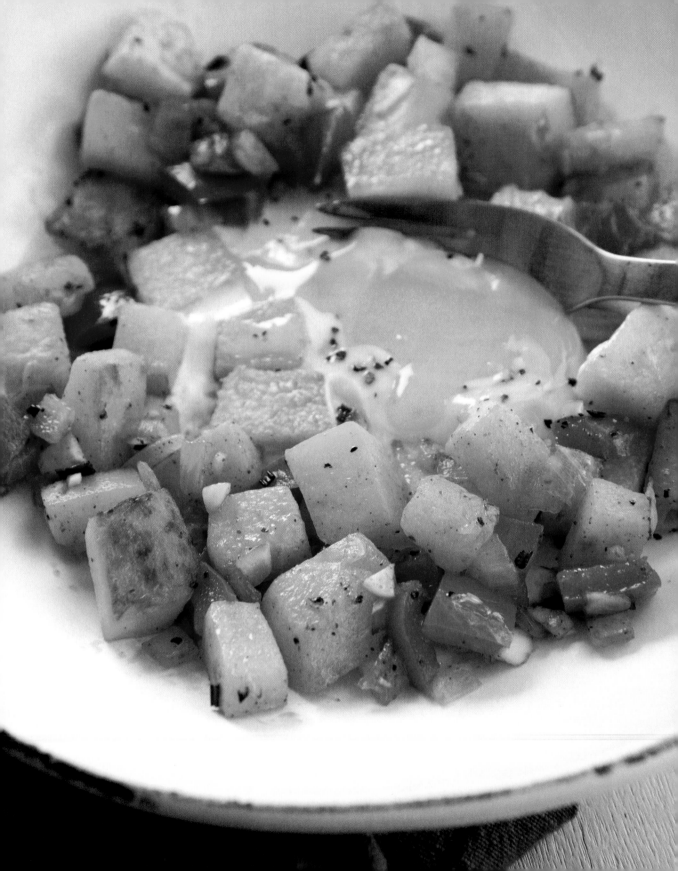

Butternut Squash Hash

Butternut squash is one of my all-time favorite ingredients. It has a beautiful orange color, is very filling, is great for heart health, and perhaps best of all, it's great for healthy skin and eyes. An ingredient that's beautiful and makes you beautiful? Yes, please!

Makes 2 servings | Serving size: 1 egg and ½ cup vegetables | Cook time: 15 minutes |
Prep time: 10 minutes

Per serving: calories 198; fat 12 g; saturated fat 3 g; fiber 2 g; protein 10 g; carbohydrates 13 g; sugar 5 g

---

½ cup ¼-inch-cubed butternut squash

Kosher salt and freshly ground black pepper

1 teaspoon olive oil

1 onion, roughly chopped

1 bell pepper, roughly chopped

½ teaspoon paprika

½ teaspoon chili powder

5 rosemary needles, minced

1 garlic clove, minced

2 large eggs

1. In the Instant Pot, combine the butternut squash, a pinch each of salt and pepper, and the olive oil. Set to "sauté, medium heat" and cook until lightly browned, about 5 minutes, stirring often to avoid burning. Add the onion and bell pepper and sauté until softened, about 5 minutes. Add the paprika, chili powder, rosemary, and garlic and toss to combine. Hit "cancel."

2. Make 2 wells in the hash and crack the eggs into the wells. Cover, choose the "egg" setting, and cook for 1 minute. Quick-release the pressure and serve.

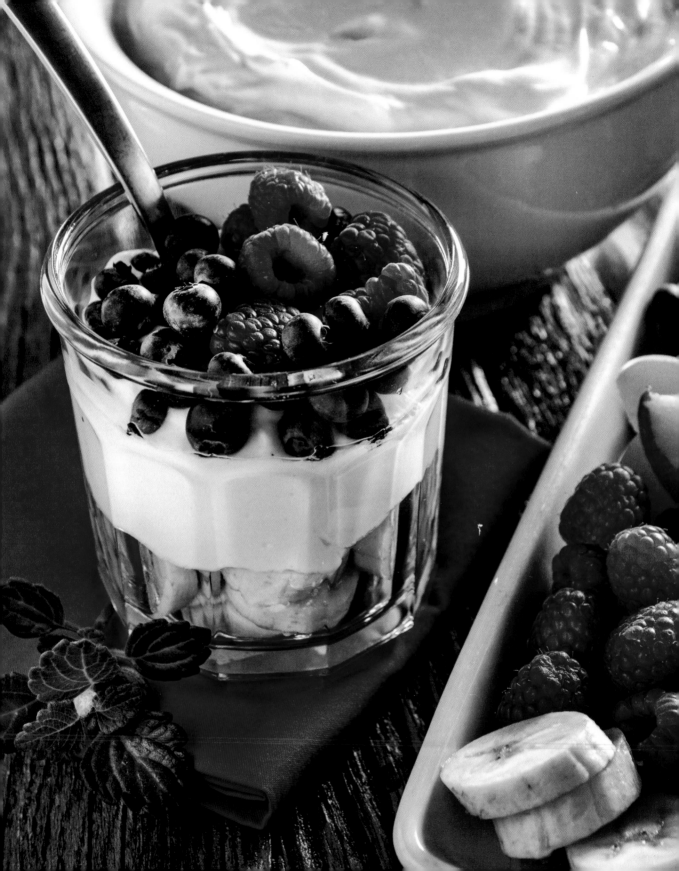

Homemade Yogurt with Fruit Topping Bar

I have one of the Instant Pot models that doesn't have a "yogurt" setting, so I had to figure out how to make yogurt without one. If you do have that feature on your Instant Pot, you can just use the manufacturer's instructions for yogurt making and refer to the topping bar suggestions below.

Makes 14 servings | Serving size: ½ cup | Cook time: 10 to 12 hours | Prep time: 3 minutes
Per serving: calories 71; fat 3 g; saturated fat 3 g; fiber 0 g; protein 5 g; carbohydrates 7 g; sugar 7 g

---

½ gallon milk (I use 2%)

2 tablespoons plain yogurt

TOPPING BAR (ALL OPTIONAL)

Sliced strawberries

Sliced banana

Blueberries

Raspberries

Peeled, diced peaches

Honey

Real maple syrup

1. Set the Instant Pot to "keep warm." Add the milk and heat uncovered for 40 minutes. Whisk, then change the setting to "sauté, medium heat." Use a thermometer to check the heat periodically; when it's reached 185°F (this will take about 15 minutes), hit "cancel" and use oven mitts to carefully remove the inner pot.

2. Let the milk cool for 40 minutes, then whisk in the yogurt. Return the inner pot to the Instant Pot, cover, close the pressure vent, and wrap the entire Instant Pot in a towel. Let the mixture sit for 8 hours or overnight.

3. Scoop the yogurt into a glass bowl, cover, and refrigerate until cold.

4. To serve, scoop ½ cup yogurt into each bowl and add your favorite toppings, or if serving a crowd, put the toppings out on the table for everyone to choose their own.

Greek Yogurt

To make thicker, Greek-style yogurt, after step 2, ladle the yogurt into a cheesecloth-lined sieve and drain for 2 to 3 hours, until thick and creamy. Proceed with step 3.

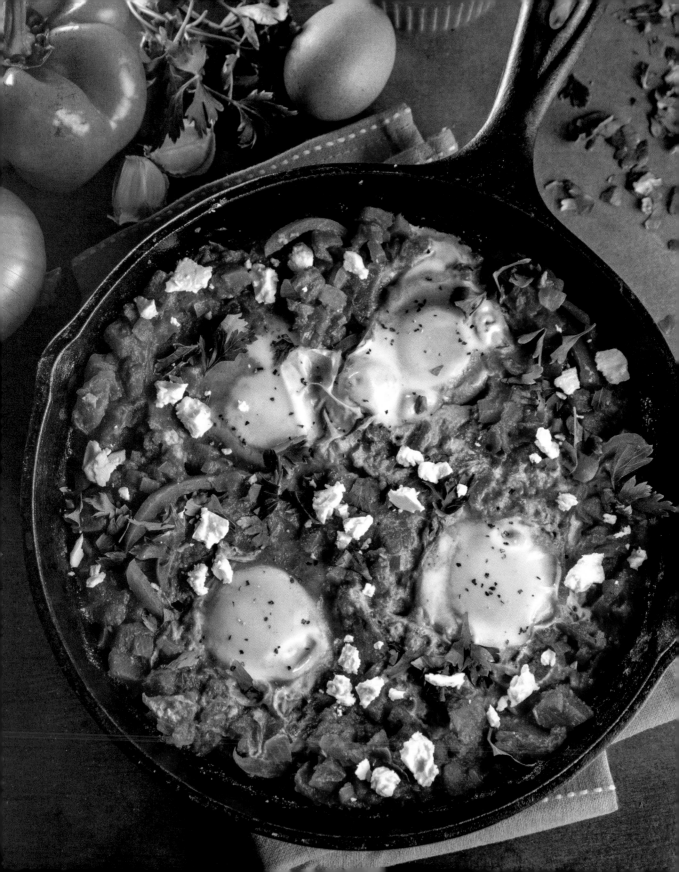

Shakshuka

This is one of my favorite brunch meals, and it's great for dinner as well. It's impressive, filling, and completely delicious. The yogurt sauce takes it to the next level, so don't skip it. And if you made the homemade Greek Yogurt (page 19), use that here!

Makes 4 servings | Serving size: 1 egg and ¼ cup yogurt sauce | Cook time: 15 to 20 minutes |
Prep time: 10 minutes
Per serving: calories 157; fat 8 g; saturated fat 3 g; fiber 5 g; protein 9 g;
carbohydrates 14 g; sugar 8 g

YOGURT SAUCE

½ cup 0% Greek yogurt

2 tablespoons chopped fresh flat-leaf parsley

¼ teaspoon garlic salt

SHAKSHUKA

1 teaspoon olive oil

1 yellow onion, finely chopped

1 red bell pepper, thinly sliced

Kosher salt

4 garlic cloves, minced

1 teaspoon ground cumin

1 teaspoon paprika

⅛ teaspoon cayenne pepper

1 (28-ounce) can chopped tomatoes

Freshly ground black pepper

4 large eggs

2 tablespoons crumbled feta cheese

¼ cup chopped fresh flat-leaf parsley

1. Make the yogurt sauce: In a small bowl, combine the ingredients. Set aside.

2. Make the *shakshuka*: In the Instant Pot, combine the olive oil, onion, bell pepper, and a pinch of salt and toss well. Set the pot to "sauté, medium heat" and cook until the vegetables start to soften, about 5 minutes. Stir often to avoid burning. Add the garlic and sauté for 2 minutes. Stir in the cumin, paprika, and cayenne. Hit "cancel."

3. Add the tomatoes and a pinch of salt and black pepper. Cover and cook on high pressure for 5 minutes.

4. Quick-release the pressure. Stir the *shakshuka* and make 4 wells in the sauce. Crack the eggs into the wells. Cover, choose the "egg" setting, and cook for 1 minute. Let the pressure release naturally for 1 minute for runny eggs or 2 to 5 minutes for firmer eggs, then quick-release the remaining pressure.

5. Sprinkle with feta and chopped parsley.

Breakfasts

21

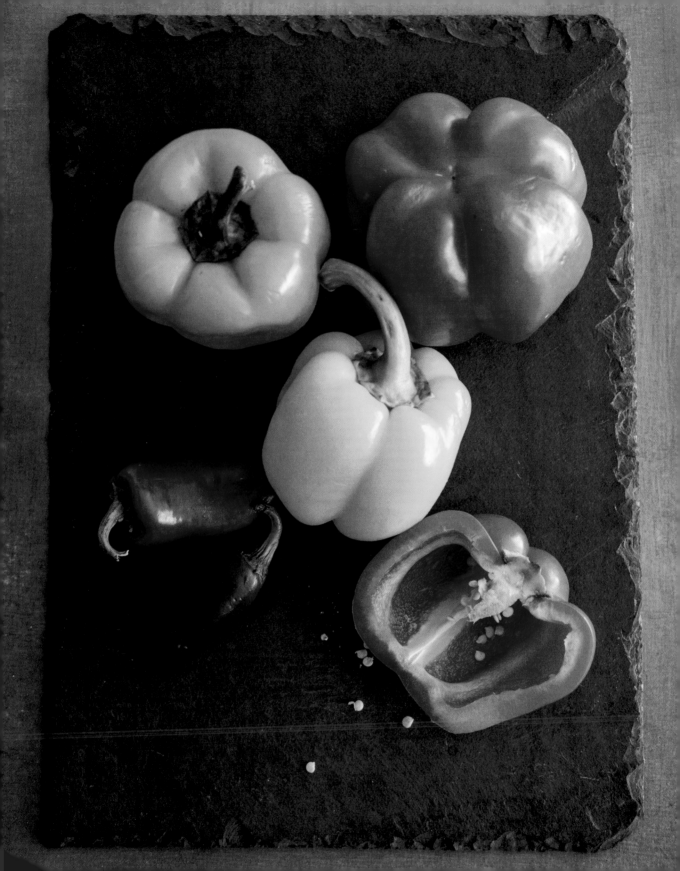

3
—

HOT LUNCHES

These filling lunch options are easy and fun to make. Some remind me of upscale versions of a school cafeteria lunch, like the Skinny Sloppy Joes (page 31) and Red Beans and Rice (page 28). Others are hot meals I love to make for myself when I'm working from home and my kiddo is at school, like the Protein Bowl (page 33).

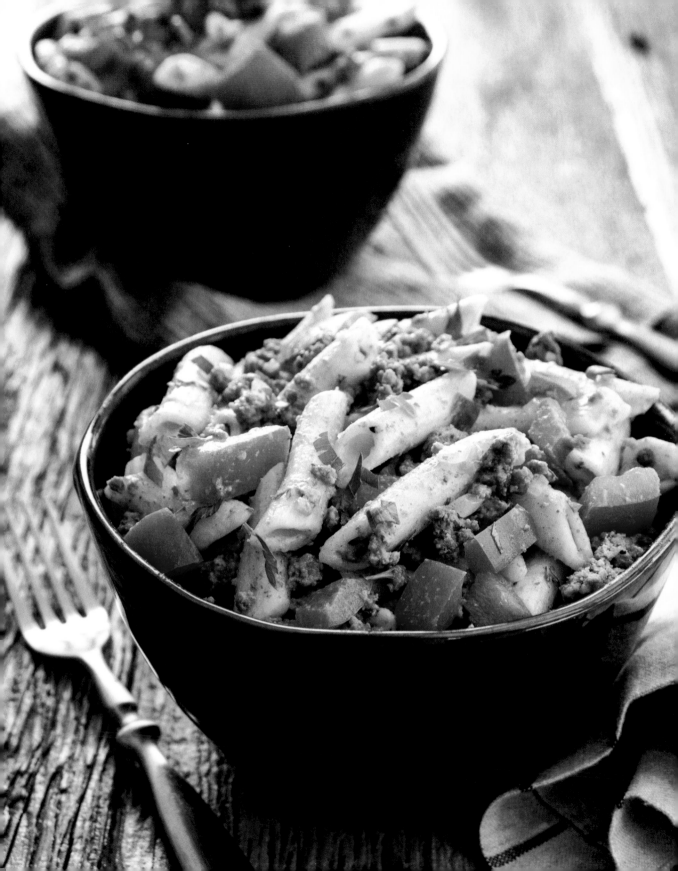

Taco Mac and Cheese

My friend Rachel called me while I was writing this cookbook and said she was making Taco Mac and Cheese for dinner. I immediately asked for the recipe, and she said, "It's your recipe!" I was confused until she explained that she had used the Skinny Mac and Cheese recipe from my first cookbook, *Lose Weight by Eating,* and added taco meat and veggies. It was sweet of her to give me credit, but I give all kudos to her for this fantastic idea. Thanks, Rach!

Makes 8 servings | Serving size: ¾ cup | Cook time: 30 minutes | Prep time: 8 minutes
Per serving: calories 271; fat 15.5 g; saturated fat 8 g; fiber 3 g; protein 19 g;
carbohydrates 25 g; sugar 8 g

---

1 teaspoon olive oil

1 red bell pepper, roughly chopped

1 onion, roughly chopped

Kosher salt and freshly ground black pepper

½ pound lean ground beef

2 tablespoons Homemade Taco Seasoning (recipe follows)

4 cups 1% milk

1 (16-ounce) box penne pasta

¾ cup grated sharp cheddar cheese

1 large tomato, cut into medium dice

¼ cup chopped fresh cilantro, parsley, or green onions (optional)

1. Set the Instant Pot to "sauté, low heat." Once it reads "hot," add the olive oil, bell pepper, onion, and a pinch each of salt and black pepper. Sauté for 5 minutes, until the vegetables start to soften.

2. Add the ground beef and taco seasoning and brown for 5 minutes. Transfer the veggies and beef to a plate.

3. Add the milk and pasta to the pot, cover, and cook for 6 minutes on high pressure.

4. Quick-release the pressure. Stir in the cheese until melted. Return the veggies and beef to the pot, add the tomato, and toss to combine. Serve hot topped with optional herbs.

Homemade Taco Seasoning

Makes ¾ cup

¼ cup chili powder

¼ cup garlic powder

2 tablespoons paprika

2 tablespoons ground cumin

2 tablespoons Italian seasoning

1 tablespoon kosher salt

1 tablespoon freshly ground black pepper

Combine all the ingredients in a jar, cover, and store for use as needed.

Italian Mac and Cheese

Okay, yes, this is very similar to baked ziti. But there are some differences:
1. You make a creamy sauce (though here it's red, not white).
2. There's no baking required.
P.S. You can trick your kids into eating anything if you call it "mac and cheese."

Makes 3 servings | Serving size: ¾ cup | Cook time: 25 minutes | Prep time: 3 minutes
Per serving: calories 378; fat 1.5 g; saturated fat 0.3 g; fiber 17 g; protein 14 g;
carbohydrates 71 g; sugar 28 g

---

1 (8-ounce) box rigatoni pasta (whole wheat if you can find it)
2½ cups Fast Marinara (page 63)
1 cup fat-free (skim) milk
⅓ cup shredded mozzarella cheese

1. In the Instant Pot, combine the pasta, marinara, and milk. Cover and cook on high pressure for 7 minutes. Let the pressure release naturally for 2 minutes, then quick-release the remaining pressure.

2. Give the mixture a good stir, add the mozzarella, and stir until the cheese is melted. Serve hot.

Red Beans and Rice

I spent some of my childhood years growing up in New Orleans, and it definitely shaped the way I experience life and food. Every Monday was red beans and rice day at my elementary school cafeteria, so one Monday, when I was missing Creole food, I pulled out my Instant Pot and made my own.

Now, I can't find andouille sausage in Boise, Idaho, so I purchased all-natural smoked sausage and was pleased to find it was a fantastic substitution. If you can find andouille sausage (and if you like spicy food), get it, but if not, just about every grocery store will have smoked sausage.

For my vegan friends, you can skip the sausage for a meatless meal!

One last note: If you have two Instant Pots (lucky!), you can make the rice in one pot and the beans in another. But making the rice on the stovetop is perfectly fine as well.

Makes 4 servings | Serving size: ½ cup red beans and ¼ cup rice | Cook time: 60 minutes |
Prep time: 10 minutes
Per serving: calories 375; fat 25.5 g; saturated fat 4.5 g; fiber 11 g; protein 21 g;
carbohydrates 30 g; sugar 1 g

---

1 tablespoon olive oil

12 ounces all-natural smoked sausage or andouille sausage, cut on the diagonal into ½-inch-thick slices

1 onion, minced

3 celery stalks, minced

6 garlic cloves, minced

2 tablespoons paprika

1 tablespoon kosher salt

1 teaspoon freshly ground black pepper

1 teaspoon cayenne pepper

1 teaspoon dried oregano

1 teaspoon dried thyme

½ teaspoon ground allspice

1 cup dried red beans

5 cups water

2 bay leaves

1 teaspoon hot sauce (preferably Crystal), plus more for serving

1 cup cooked rice (try it in your Instant Pot!)

Chopped fresh flat-leaf parsley (optional), for serving

Sliced green onions (optional), for serving

1. Set the Instant Pot to "sauté, medium heat." Once it reads "hot," add the olive oil and sausage and cook, stirring occassionally, for 3 to 5 minutes or until browned. Remove the sausage to a plate.

2. Add the onion and celery and sauté until soft, about 5 minutes. Add the garlic, paprika, salt, black pepper, cayenne, oregano, thyme, and allspice. Hit "cancel."

3. Add the beans, water, bay leaves, hot sauce, and sausage (including any juices on the plate). Cover and cook on high pressure for 45 minutes.

4. Let the pressure release naturally; this will allow the beans to continue cooking. When the pressure is fully released, test the beans by gently smashing one. I like my beans to have a bit of bite to them—al dente, if you like—but if you prefer a softer bean, cover, and cook on high pressure for 10 minutes longer, then quick-release the pressure.

5. Serve the beans in bowls over a scoop of rice and topped with a sprinkling of parsley and green onions (if using).

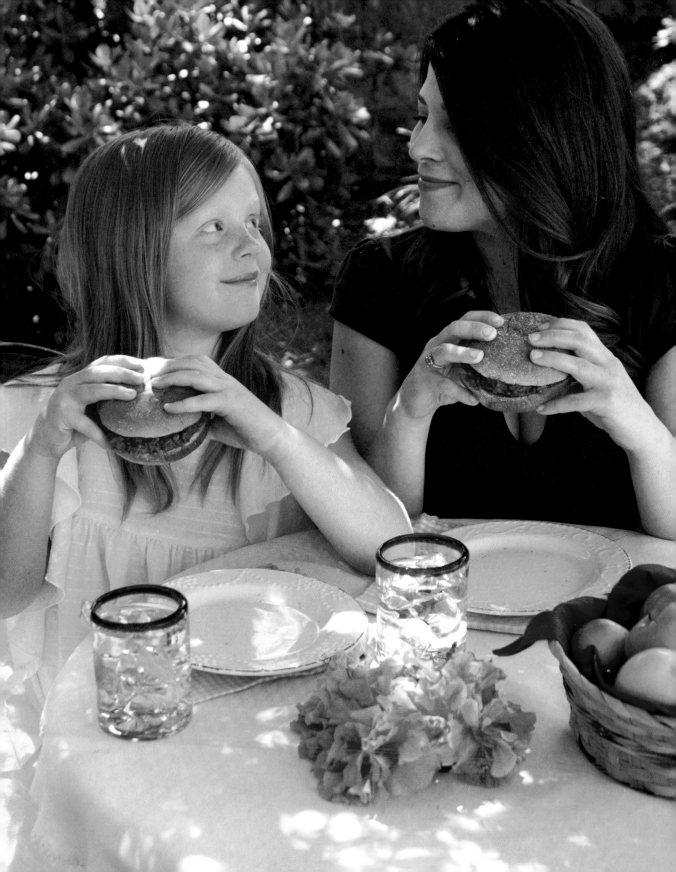

Skinny Sloppy Joes

I gave the recipe for these sloppy joes from my first cookbook, *Lose Weight by Eating*, an Instant Pot makeover. They're packed full of vegetables—in fact, the meat mixture is half vegetables! Yes, you read that right—this recipe is 50 percent veggies. It's a well-rounded meal, with veggies, lean protein, and whole grains. Just don't tell the kids—the vegetables are so well hidden that they'll never notice unless you let the cat out of the bag.

Makes 6 servings | Serving size: 1 sandwich | Cook time: 35 minutes | Prep time: 8 minutes

Per serving: calories 347; fat 9.5 g; saturated fat 2 g; fiber 9 g; protein 21 g;
carbohydrates 45 g; sugar 19 g

---

1 teaspoon olive oil

1 onion, minced

1 red bell pepper, minced

Kosher salt and freshly ground black
  pepper

3 garlic cloves, minced

1 pound lean ground turkey

1 carrot, grated

1 (6-ounce) can tomato paste

1 (16-ounce) can tomato sauce

1 tablespoon Dijon mustard

1 tablespoon pure maple syrup

1 tablespoon balsamic vinegar

1 tablespoon paprika

1 teaspoon chili powder

6 whole wheat burger buns

1. In the Instant Pot, combine the olive oil, onion, and bell pepper and set the pot to "sauté, medium heat."

Sprinkle lightly with salt and black pepper and sauté for 5 minutes, until the vegetables start to soften. Add the garlic and cook for 2 minutes. Add the turkey and carrot and brown for 5 minutes, breaking up the meat as it cooks. Add the tomato paste, tomato sauce, mustard, maple syrup, balsamic vinegar, paprika, and chili powder. Stir to combine.

2. Cover and cook on high pressure for 3 minutes. Let the pressure release naturally. At this point I leave it on "warm" and walk away until mealtime, but you can uncover and serve on the buns right away. The first time I made this I left it on "warm" for 3 hours while I held a Girl Scout meeting—it's a great recipe for making and walking away!

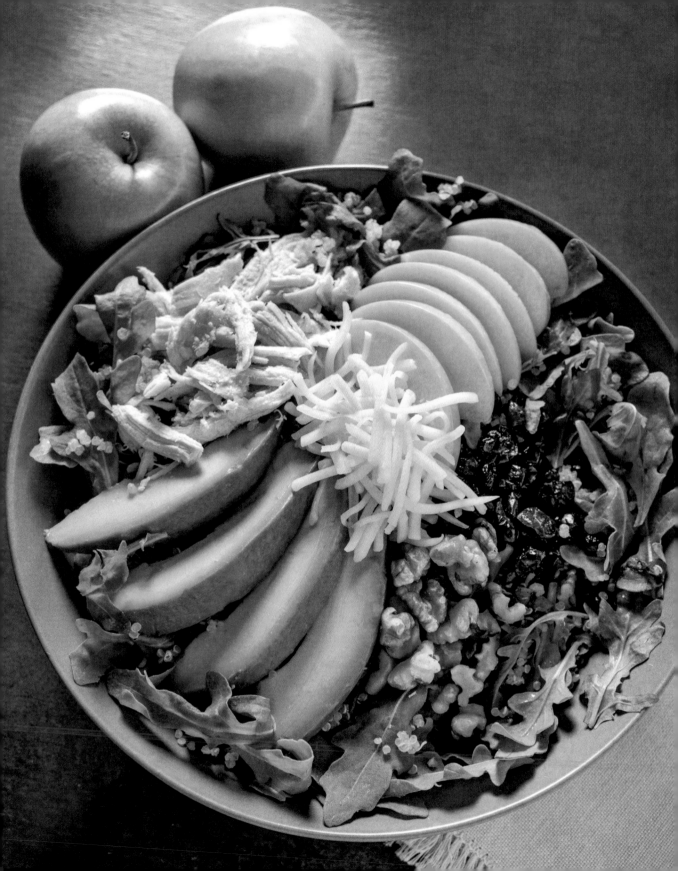

Protein Bowl

Protein bowls are all the rage; I've seen them on menus all over town. I felt out of the loop, so one day I called my good friend Heidi and asked her to meet me at one of these places for lunch. I ordered their signature protein bowl and was blown away by how delicious it was, and how fast they were able to put it together.

Makes 4 servings | Serving size: 1 bowl | Cook time: 20 minutes | Prep time: 8 minutes
Per serving: calories 391; fat 16.5 g; saturated fat 3.5 g; fiber 8 g; protein 34 g;
carbohydrates 27 g; sugar 6 g

DRESSING

Juice of 1 orange

1 tablespoon apple cider vinegar

2 garlic cloves, minced

1 teaspoon extra-virgin olive oil

1 tablespoon Dijon mustard

Kosher salt and freshly ground black pepper

PROTEIN BOWL

½ cup uncooked quinoa, rinsed

½ cup water

2 boneless, skinless chicken breasts

Kosher salt and freshly ground black pepper

4 cups mixed greens

1 green apple, cored and thinly sliced

1 avocado, thinly sliced

2 tablespoons chopped walnuts

2 tablespoons dried cranberries

¼ cup shredded Monterey Jack cheese

1. Make the dressing: In a small bowl, whisk together the ingredients. Set aside.

2. Make the protein bowl: In the Instant Pot, combine the quinoa and water. Add the rack and the steamer basket to the pot and place the chicken breasts in the steamer basket. Sprinkle with salt and pepper. Cover and cook on high pressure for 12 minutes.

3. Quick-release the pressure. Carefully lift the steamer basket (use oven mitts) out of the pot. Transfer the chicken to a cutting board and shred or chop it into bite-size pieces.

4. Transfer the quinoa to a large bowl. Add the greens and pour the dressing on top. Toss to coat the lettuce evenly.

5. Divide the lettuce among 4 bowls. Divide the chicken, apple, avocado, walnuts, and cranberries among the bowls, assembling the ingredients individually around the sides of the bowl like a clock. Sprinkle the cheese in the center of each bowl and serve.

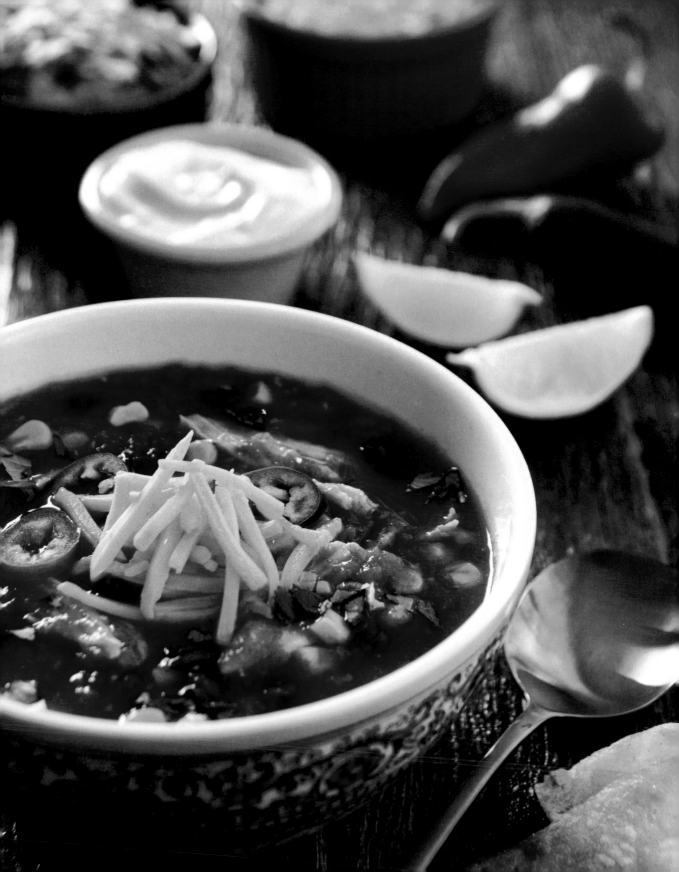

Chicken Enchilada Soup

We love enchiladas in our home. My daughter called them enchi-la-las for a long time, so we still have fun with it and call this enchi-la-la soup.

This soup is great with or without the toppings, but a topping bar will impress both family members and dinner guests.

Makes 4 servings │ Serving size: 1 cup │ Cook time: 55 minutes │ Prep time: 8 minutes
Per serving: calories 262; fat 3.5 g; saturated fat 0.5 g; fiber 15 g; protein 15 g;
carbohydrates 45 g; sugar 8 g

1 yellow onion, minced

1 jalapeño, seeds and ribs removed, minced

4 garlic cloves, minced

1 teaspoon olive oil

Kosher salt and freshly ground black
  pepper

1 (28-ounce) can crushed tomatoes

½ teaspoon ground allspice

1 boneless, skinless chicken breast, cut into
  ¼-inch cubes

1½ cups chicken broth

½ cup frozen corn

1 (16-ounce) can black beans, drained and
  rinsed

OPTIONAL TOPPINGS

Shredded cheddar cheese

Chopped fresh cilantro

Crumbled tortilla chips

Greek yogurt (tastes like sour cream!)

Hot sauce

Chopped fresh or pickled jalapeños

1. In the Instant Pot, combine the onion, jalapeño, garlic, olive oil, and a pinch each of salt and pepper and mix together. Set the pot to "sauté, medium heat" and cook for 10 minutes, until the vegetables have softened, stirring often to avoid burning.

2. Transfer the mixture to a blender, add the tomatoes and allspice, and blend until smooth.

3. Return the blended vegetables to the pot and add the chicken, broth, corn, and beans. Cover, choose the "soup" setting, and cook for 25 minutes.

4. Let the pressure release naturally for 10 minutes, then quick-release the remaining pressure. Serve with toppings, if desired.

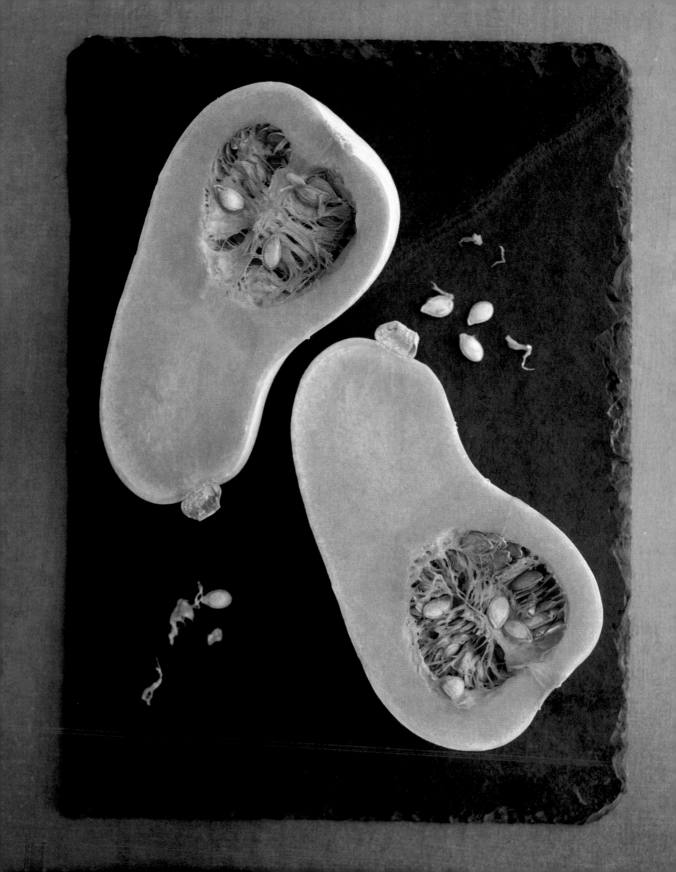

4

ONE-POT DINNERS

I'm not a fan of making a big mess in the kitchen, so I really love one-pot meals! These are easy and range from comfort food like Chicken and Dumplings (page 45) and Skinny "Crack" Chicken (page 49) to more elegant meals, like Cassoulet (page 41) and Bruschetta Chicken (page 51), that you can make for a dinner party.

Beef Bourguignon

This traditional French stew usually takes about 3 hours . . . but not in the Instant Pot! Here it's just 1 hour from start to finish, including coming to pressure.

I cut the calories by cutting down on the wine and removing the brandy from the recipe. I can't tell the difference, and considering that cooking under pressure does not burn off the alcohol at the same rate, it's an important cut to make! Don't fret, we sauté off any remaining alcohol in the end; just don't skip that step unless you want a boozy dinner! If you want to skip the wine altogether, just use 2 cups of beef broth and add an extra tablespoon of tomato paste.

Makes 4 servings | Serving size: 1¼ cups | Cook time: 60 minutes | Prep time: 15 minutes
Per serving: calories 298; fat 12.5 g; saturated fat 2.5 g; fiber 3 g; protein 26 g;
carbohydrates 19 g; sugar 6 g

---

1 pound beef chuck, cut into ½-inch cubes
1 tablespoon all-purpose flour
Kosher salt and freshly ground black pepper
1 tablespoon olive oil
2 onions, roughly chopped
3 carrots, cut on the diagonal into ¼-inch-thick slices
2 celery stalks, cut on the diagonal into ¼-inch-thick slices
2 garlic cloves, chopped
1 cup sliced white mushrooms
1 cup dry red wine
1 cup beef broth
1 tablespoon tomato paste
2 fresh thyme sprigs
2 tablespoons cornstarch
½ cup frozen pearl onions, thawed
Chopped fresh parsley (optional)

1. In a large bowl, toss together the beef, flour, and a sprinkling of salt and pepper.

2. Set the Instant Pot to "sauté, medium heat." Once it reads "hot," add ½ tablespoon of the olive oil and, working in batches, brown the beef in the hot pot, transferring it to a plate as you finish. Add the remaining ½ tablespoon of olive oil, onions, carrots, celery, and a light sprinkling of salt to the pot and sauté the vegetables for 5 minutes, until softened. Add the garlic and mushrooms and sauté for 2 minutes. Hit "cancel."

3. Add the wine and scrape the bottom of the pot to loosen up any browned bits, then add the broth and mix in the tomato paste. Return the

beef to the pot and mix to combine. Place the thyme sprigs on top of the stew. Cover and cook on high pressure for 30 minutes.

4. Let the pressure release naturally for 10 minutes, then quick-release the remaining pressure. Pluck out the thyme stems (the leaves will most likely have fallen off).

5. Transfer ¼ cup of the broth to a bowl and whisk it with the cornstarch. Return the cornstarch mixture to the pot and mix well. Add the pearl onions. Set the pot to "sauté, high heat" and cook for 5 minutes, to burn off any alcohol and cook the pearl onions. Taste and add more salt and pepper as needed.

6. Serve in bowls and top with parsley if desired. This stew gets better the second day, so save the leftovers or make a double batch (same cooking time!) to enjoy the leftovers all week.

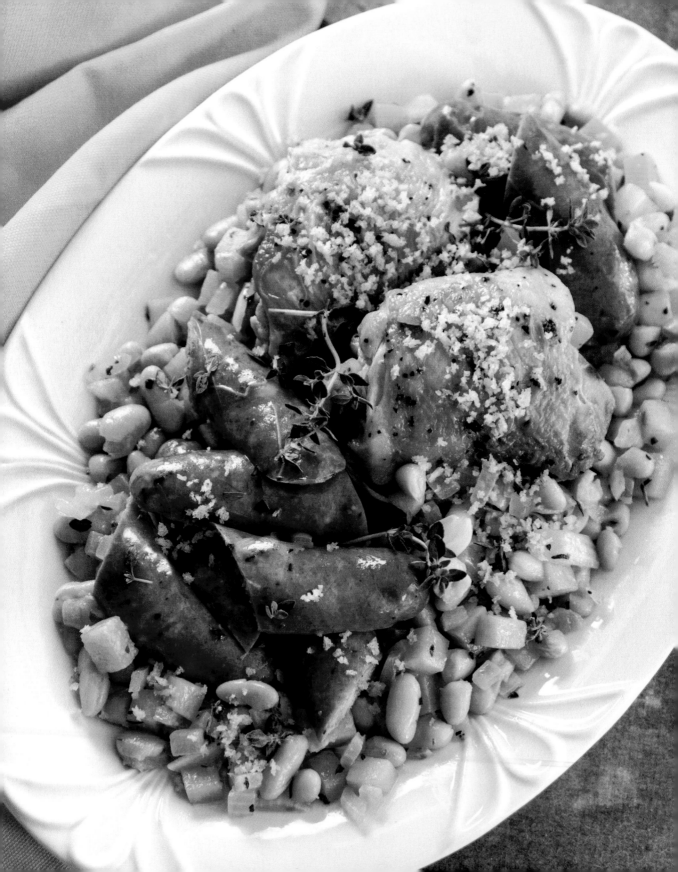

Cassoulet

Here's one of those dishes that you can basically use any cut of chicken in. I prefer bone-in chicken thighs, as the bones and the dark meat add a complexity that you don't get with a boneless, skinless chicken breast . . . but if that's all you have, by all means, use it!

I originally made this with gluten-free bread crumbs for a dinner guest who is gluten intolerant, and it came out great. Just make sure to get panko-style bread crumbs should you choose to opt for gluten-free.

Makes 2 servings | Serving size: 1 piece of chicken, ½ sausage, and ½ cup beans |
Cook time: 45 minutes | Prep time: 8 minutes
Per serving: calories 615; fat 40 g; saturated fat 11 g; fiber 7 g; protein 39 g;
carbohydrates 28 g; sugar 6 g

---

1 teaspoon olive oil
Kosher salt and freshly ground black
    pepper
2 bone-in chicken thighs
1 cup water
1 (¼-pound) smoked sausage link,
    halved crosswise
1 onion, finely chopped
1 cup ½-inch-cubed butternut squash
2 garlic cloves, minced
1 (16-ounce) can cannellini beans,
    drained and rinsed
1 tablespoon Italian seasoning
1 teaspoon ground thyme
1 teaspoon butter
¼ cup panko bread crumbs

1. Set the Instant Pot to "sauté, medium heat." Once it reads "hot," add ½ teaspoon of the olive oil. Sprinkle salt and pepper over the chicken, then add the chicken to the pot skin side down and brown for 3 to 5 minutes, until browned on that side.

2. Flip the chicken, add the water, and hit "cancel." Cover and cook on high pressure for 20 minutes. Quick-release the pressure and transfer the chicken to a plate. Transfer the broth to a bowl or large glass measuring cup.

3. Set the pot to "sauté, medium heat" and add the remaining ½ teaspoon olive oil. Add the sausage and brown for 3 minutes on each side, then transfer to the plate with the chicken.

4. Add the onion and squash and sauté for 5 minutes, stirring often to avoid burning. Add the garlic and cook for 2 minutes. Hit "cancel."

5. Add the beans, Italian seasoning, thyme, and reserved chicken broth and stir to combine. Add the chicken and sausage, cover, and cook on high pressure for 5 minutes.

6. Meanwhile, in a skillet, melt the butter over low heat. Toss in the panko and toast until golden brown. Remove from the heat to avoid burning.

7. Back at the Instant Pot, quick-release the pressure. Transfer the chicken, sausage, and beans to a serving platter, top with toasted bread crumbs, and serve.

Fast Fajitas

Truth be told, fajitas are fast no matter how you cook them. These are slightly faster than the average fajita recipe, but the real difference is you can walk away from them as they cook. So, you can get them started when you come home from work, then walk away without worrying that they will burn.

Makes 4 servings | Serving size: ½ cup fajitas and 2 tortillas | Cook time: 20 minutes |
Prep time: 8 minutes
Per serving: calories 219; fat 4 g; saturated fat 1 g; fiber 4 g; protein 17 g;
carbohydrates 30 g; sugar 3 g

---

1 teaspoon olive oil

1 yellow onion, thinly sliced

1 red bell pepper, thinly sliced

2 jalapeños, seeds and ribs removed, thinly sliced

Kosher salt and freshly ground black pepper

1 boneless, skinless chicken breast, thinly sliced

1 teaspoon garlic powder

1 teaspoon chili powder

½ teaspoon cayenne pepper

1 teaspoon Italian seasoning

Juice of 2 limes

¾ cup water

8 corn tortillas

OPTIONAL TOPPINGS

Shredded sharp cheddar cheese

Chopped fresh cilantro

Sliced jalapeños

Greek yogurt (tastes just like sour cream)

Hot sauce or salsa

1. Set the Instant Pot to "sauté, medium heat." Once it reads "hot," add the oil, onion, bell pepper, and jalapeños. Sprinkle lightly with salt and black pepper and sauté for 5 minutes, until the vegetables are softened.

2. Add the chicken, garlic powder, chili powder, cayenne, and Italian seasoning and mix to combine. Hit "cancel."

3. Add the lime juice and water. Cover and cook on high pressure for 2 minutes. At this point you can walk away and make yourself a margarita. Quick-release the pressure. Remove the fajitas to a plate.

4. Set the pot to "sauté, high heat" and simmer until the liquid reduces by half, about 3 to 5 minutes. Return the fajitas to the pot, hit "cancel," and toss the fajitas and sauce together. Serve with the tortillas and optional toppings.

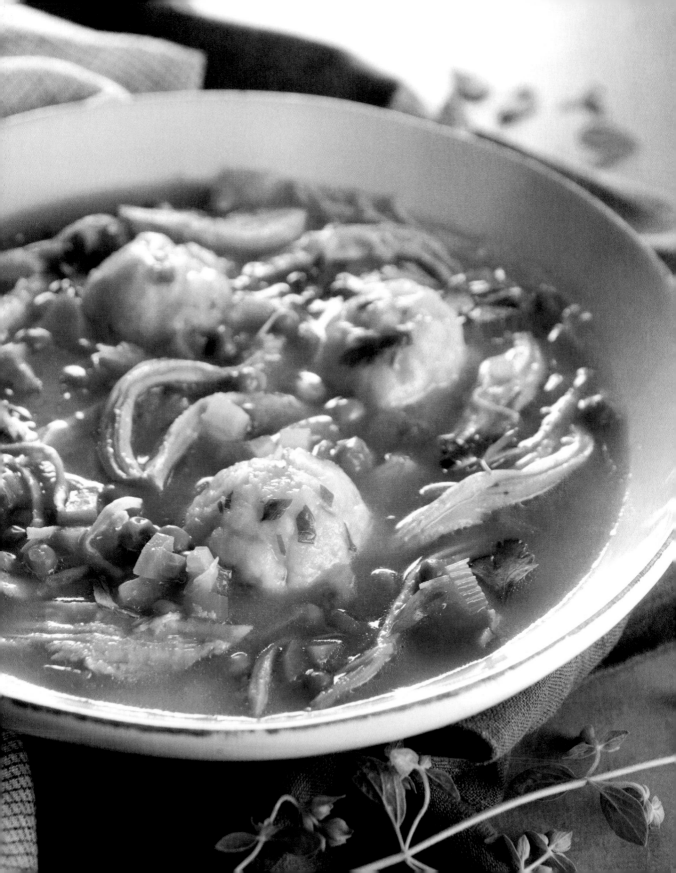

Chicken and Dumplings

Two days before my daughter, Sophia, and I were to leave for my first appearance on *Today,* we both got sick. It was just a cold, but a bad one, with headaches, aches and pains, runny noses, and nasty coughs. I was terrified that I would lose my voice or she would feel too awful to enjoy her first trip to New York. So, I made this soup, and it cured us! I'm not kidding. In fact, I'm typing this on the plane on my way to the *Today* appearance, and I feel great! Nervous, but great.

Make this for your sick kids, and yourself, and feel better fast!

Makes 4 servings | Serving size: 1¼ cups | Cook time: 35 minutes | Prep time: 15 minutes
Per serving: calories 334; fat 5.5 g; saturated fat 1 g; fiber 3 g; protein 32 g;
carbohydrates 38 g; sugar 8 g

---

2 boneless, skinless chicken breasts

Kosher salt and freshly ground black pepper

1 teaspoon garlic powder

1 teaspoon onion powder

1½ cups water

1 teaspoon olive oil

1 yellow onion, minced

2 carrots, minced

2 celery stalks, minced

2 garlic cloves, minced

½ cup unsweetened almond milk (any unsweetened milk will work)

1 teaspoon dried oregano

¾ cup frozen peas

DUMPLINGS

1 cup all-purpose flour

½ cup unsweetened almond milk (any unsweetened milk will work)

1 teaspoon kosher salt

1 teaspoon baking powder

1 teaspoon chopped fresh flat-leaf parsley

2 tablespoons cornstarch

1 tablespoon chopped fresh flat-leaf parsley, for garnish

1. Sprinkle the chicken breasts lightly with salt and pepper and add them to the Instant Pot with the garlic powder, onion powder, and water. Cover and cook on high pressure for 20 minutes. Quick-release the pressure. Transfer the chicken to a plate and the broth to a heatproof bowl or large glass measuring cup. When cool enough to handle, shred the chicken with 2 forks.

2. Set the Instant Pot to "sauté, medium heat." Once it reads "hot," add the olive oil, onion, carrots,

celery, and garlic and sauté for 3 minutes. Add the chicken, reserved broth, milk, oregano, peas, and a pinch of salt and pepper. Hit "cancel." Cover and cook on high pressure for 10 minutes.

3. Meanwhile, make the dumplings: In a medium bowl, combine the flour, milk, salt, baking powder, and parsley and mix with a wooden spoon until just combined. Set aside until the Instant Pot turns off.

4. Quick-release the pressure. Transfer ¼ cup of the liquid to a small bowl. Add the cornstarch to the bowl and whisk well. Pour the cornstarch mixture into the pot and mix to combine.

5. Set the pot to "sauté, low heat" and drop in the dumpling dough in balls the size of Ping-Pong balls. Simmer for 5 to 7 minutes, until the dumplings float.

6. Serve garnished with fresh parsley.

Chicken Thighs and Orzo

I love, love, love Mediterranean food . . . so flavorful and healthy! When my food stylist asked what I wanted on the cover of this book, it had to be this colorful and impressive dish. Serve it at a dinner party with a crisp salad and some hummus and pita, and your guests will be very happy.

Makes 4 servings | Serving size: 1 chicken thigh and ⅓ cup orzo | Cook time: 40 minutes |
Prep time: 12 minutes
Per serving: calories 208; fat 9 g; saturated fat 2.5 g; fiber 2 g; protein 21 g;
carbohydrates 12 g; sugar 4 g

4 bone-in, skin-on chicken thighs
Kosher salt and freshly ground black pepper
1 teaspoon olive oil
1 yellow onion, minced
1 red bell pepper, minced
4 garlic cloves, minced
1 medium Roma (plum) tomato, finely
　chopped
8 Kalamata olives, quartered
1 teaspoon minced fresh dill
½ cup uncooked orzo
Juice of 1 lemon
1 cup water

YOGURT TOPPING
½ cup 0% Greek yogurt
¼ teaspoon garlic salt
½ teaspoon minced fresh dill
1 teaspoon chopped fresh flat-leaf parsley,
　plus more for garnish

1. Sprinkle the chicken with salt and pepper. Set the Instant Pot to "sauté, medium heat." Once it reads "hot," add the olive oil. Add the chicken skin side down and brown for 5 minutes. Flip the chicken, add the onion, bell pepper, and garlic, and sauté for 5 minutes, until the vegetables start to soften.

2. Transfer the chicken to a plate. Add the tomato, olives, dill, orzo, lemon juice, and water to the pot. Stir to combine. Return the chicken to the pot, skin side up. Cover and cook on high pressure for 10 minutes.

3. Make the yogurt topping: In a small bowl, combine ingredients and set aside.

4. Let the pressure release naturally for 10 minutes, then quick-release the remaining pressure. If the sauce is watery, remove the chicken to a plate and cook the sauce on "sauté, low heat" for 2 to 5 minutes, stirring often to ensure that nothing burns.

5. Serve the chicken and orzo topped with the yogurt and more parsley.

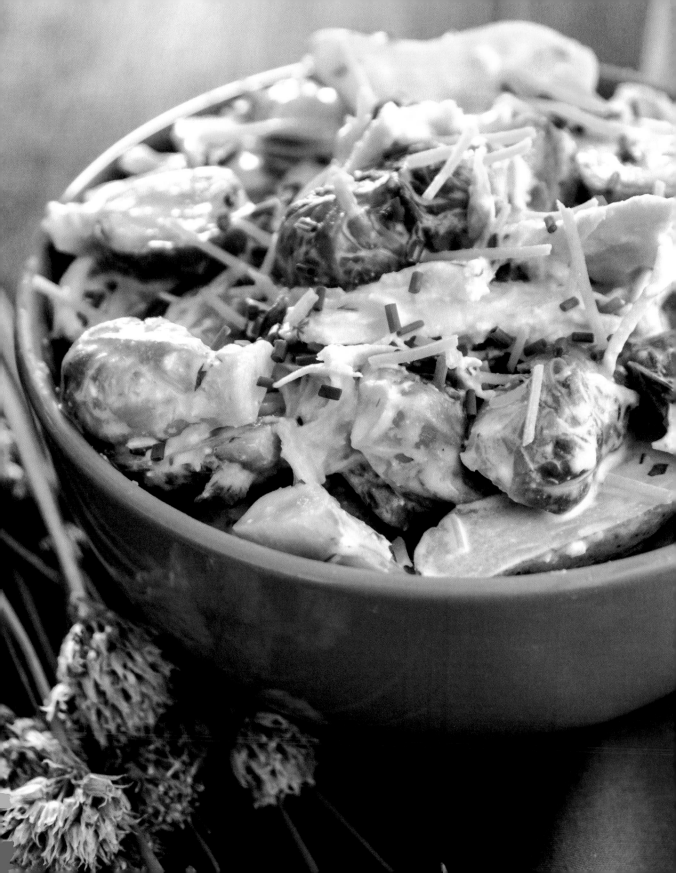

Skinny "Crack" Chicken

When researching for this cookbook, I kept coming across recipes for "crack" chicken. Everyone was talking about this dish and seemed to love it, but I was shocked at the calorie-heavy ingredients.

I had to come up with a healthier version, so you can still enjoy this decadent dish and avoid packing on the pounds. This is just as addictive as the full-calorie version, but you won't feel so guilty about enjoying it weekly.

Makes 4 servings | Serving size: 1 cup | Cook time: 25 minutes | Prep time: 15 minutes
Per serving: calories 349; fat 12.5 g; saturated fat 6 g; fiber 3 g; protein 43 g;
carbohydrates 16 g; sugar 2 g

½ pound fingerling potatoes, halved crosswise

½ pound Brussels sprouts, trimmed, dark outer leaves removed, halved through the stem

1 pound boneless, skinless chicken breast

2 ounces Neufchâtel cheese (you'll find it next to the cream cheese at the store)

½ teaspoon garlic salt

1 tablespoon minced fresh chives

1 teaspoon minced fresh dill

1 teaspoon chopped fresh flat-leaf parsley

¾ cup water

¼ cup shredded sharp cheddar cheese

1. In the Instant Pot, combine the potatoes, Brussels sprouts, chicken, Neufchâtel cheese, garlic salt, chives, dill, parsley, and water. Cover and cook on high pressure for 15 minutes.

2. Quick-release the pressure. Remove the chicken to a plate. Shred the chicken with two forks and return it to the pot. Mix in the cheddar cheese and serve.

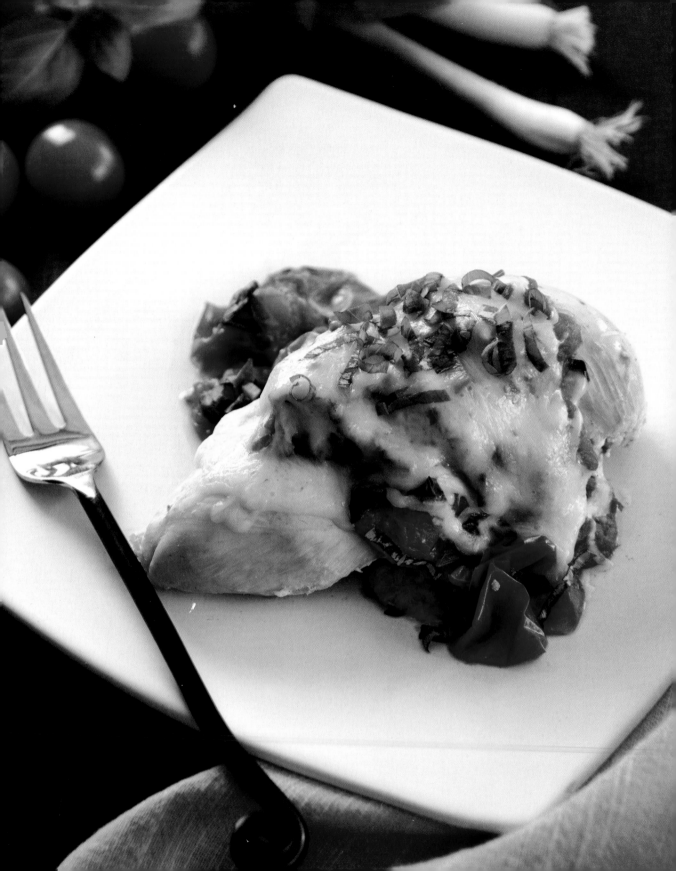

Bruschetta Chicken

The idea behind this fast meal is that you can stop by the grocery store on the way home from work, dump everything in the Instant Pot when you get home, and be eating within the hour.

I love bruschetta and often make it with big, plump tomatoes (see page 69), but I wanted to make it even easier for you. So simply buy one of those little cartons of cherry tomatoes and call it a day.

Makes 2 servings | Serving size: 1 chicken breast and ⅓ cup bruschetta topping |
Cook time: 25 minutes | Prep time: 5 minutes
Per serving: calories 399; fat 6.5 g; saturated fat 2 g; fiber 3 g; protein 60 g;
carbohydrates 25 g; sugar 19 g

---

10 ounces cherry tomatoes

2 garlic cloves, minced

1 green onion, sliced

½ cup water

2 boneless, skinless chicken breasts

Kosher salt and freshly ground black pepper

¼ cup chopped fresh basil leaves

¼ cup shredded mozzarella cheese

1. In the Instant Pot, combine the tomatoes, garlic, green onion, and water.

2. Put the rack and steamer basket in the pot. Place the chicken in the steamer basket and sprinkle with salt and pepper. Cover and cook on high pressure for 10 minutes.

3. Let the pressure release naturally. Carefully lift the steamer basket (use oven mitts) out of the pot. Place the chicken out on two plates. Remove the rack from the pot and stir the basil into the tomato mixture. Ladle the hot tomato mixture over the chicken breasts.

4. Immediately sprinkle the mozzarella over everything, letting it melt a bit, and serve.

Chicken Tortilla Soup

While I was testing recipes for this book, a good friend got sick and had to cancel our lunch date. Well, I'm a cookbook author, so naturally I had to cook for him.

This recipe for tortilla soup is in my first cookbook, *Lose Weight by Eating,* and I wondered if it could be done in an Instant Pot. Guess what? It can be! I changed it up a bit and made some gluten-free modifications to suit my friend's needs, then I "drive-by"-bombed his front door with soup. Which sounds as if I threw it at the door, but sadly I just left it with a note. There's always next time (wink, wink).

Makes 6 servings | Serving size: 1 cup | Cook time: 40 minutes | Prep time: 13 minutes
Per serving: calories 114; fat 3 g; saturated fat 1 g; fiber 3 g; protein 11 g;
carbohydrates 11 g; sugar 6 g

---

1 teaspoon olive oil

1 yellow onion, roughly chopped

1 red bell pepper, roughly chopped

Kosher salt and freshly ground black
   pepper

3 garlic cloves, minced

2 jalapeños, seeded and minced

4 large tomatoes, cut into rough
   chunks

1 cup water

2 tablespoons chili powder

½ teaspoon ground cumin

1 tablespoon dried oregano

1 carrot, halved lengthwise
   and cut into ½-inch-thick
   half-moons

1 boneless, skinless chicken breast

¼ cup frozen corn kernels

½ cup milk (I used 1% but any will do)

TOPPINGS (OPTIONAL)

Corn tortilla chips

Diced avocado

Fresh cilantro

Shredded sharp cheddar cheese

1. Set the Instant Pot to "sauté, medium heat." Once it reads "hot," add the olive oil. Stir in the onion and bell pepper, sprinkle with salt and black pepper, and sauté for about 5 minutes, until the vegetables start to soften. Add the garlic and jalapeños and sauté for 2 minutes.

2. In a blender, combine the tomatoes and water and blend until smooth.

3. Add the chili powder, cumin, oregano, and carrot to the pot and cook for 1 to 2 minutes, until the spices become fragrant. Add the

tomato sauce, chicken, and corn. Cover and cook on high pressure for 20 minutes.

4. Quick-release the pressure. Transfer the chicken to a plate. Set the pot to "sauté, medium heat" and add the milk.

5. Shred the chicken and return it to the soup. Simmer for 10 minutes, then serve with toppings, if desired.

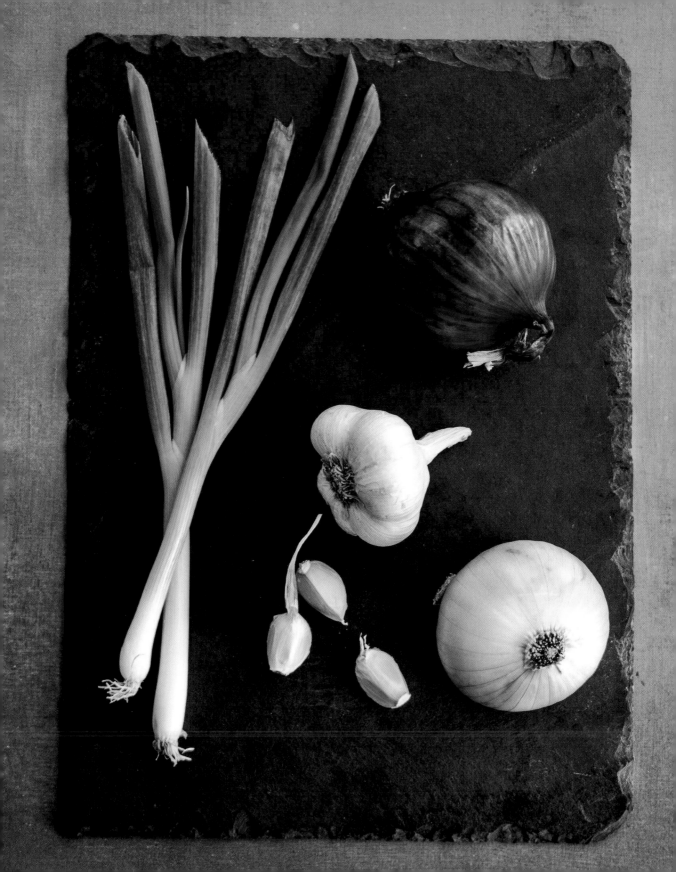

5
MAIN DISHES

These main dishes go great with your favorite salads and sides (check out the sides in the next chapter, page 67). I love to pair the "Rotisserie" Chicken (page 56) with the Bruschetta (page 69) and serve the French Onion Chicken (page 61) with the Rosemary Fingerling Potatoes (page 77).

"Rotisserie" Chicken

My preferred method for cooking chicken will always be roasting, but that can be daunting and very time consuming. You won't get crispy skin on this Instant Pot version, but you will get perfectly cooked, juicy chicken that your family will rave about.

Makes 8 servings | Serving size: 4 ounces of chicken | Cook time: 60 minutes |
Prep time: 10 minutes
Per serving: calories 336; fat 9.5 g; saturated fat 2 g; fiber 0 g; protein 58 g;
carbohydrates 2 g; sugar 1 g

---

1 tablespoon olive oil

1 (5-pound) chicken

2 garlic cloves, chopped

1 yellow onion, cut into ½-inch-thick rings

1 teaspoon chili powder

1 teaspoon ground cumin

1 teaspoon paprika

½ teaspoon kosher salt

½ teaspoon freshly ground black pepper

1 cup water

1. Set the Instant Pot to "sauté, medium heat" and add the olive oil. Once it reads "hot," add the chicken, breast side down. Brown the chicken for 8 to 10 minutes, moving it as needed to brown it on all sides.

2. Remove the chicken from the pot. Add the garlic and onion and sauté for 5 minutes, until softened.

3. Meanwhile, in a bowl, combine the chili powder, cumin, paprika, salt, and black pepper. Sprinkle the rub all over the chicken.

4. Pour the water into the pot and set the rack inside. Lay the chicken on the rack breast side up, cover, and cook on high pressure for 30 minutes.

5. Let the pressure release naturally for 10 minutes, then quick-release the remaining pressure. Transfer the chicken to a cutting board. Let rest for 15 minutes before carving.

BBQ Chicken

This recipe may have a lot of ingredients, but don't let that turn you off! It's a simple dump-and-cook meal: Just add everything to the pot and cook. Sometimes I make extra BBQ sauce (I just cook it in there with the chicken) and store it for other recipes.

Makes 2 or 4 servings | Serving size: 1 piece of chicken (1 breast or 1 thigh)
Cook time: 35 minutes | Prep time: 5 minutes
Per serving: calories 392; fat 9 g; saturated fat 2 g; fiber 3 g; protein 56 g;
carbohydrates 15 g; sugar 8 g

1 teaspoon olive oil

1 shallot or ½ red onion, finely chopped

1 garlic clove, minced

⅛ teaspoon kosher salt

1 cup dry red wine

¼ cup tomato paste

2 tablespoons chili powder

1 tablespoon paprika

1 tablespoon Dijon mustard

1 tablespoon red wine vinegar

1 tablespoon Worcestershire sauce

1 chipotle in adobo sauce, minced

1 teaspoon pure maple syrup

2 bone-in chicken breasts or 4 bone-in chicken thighs

1. In the Instant Pot, combine everything but the chicken. Add the chicken and turn the pieces in the sauce to coat all over. Cover and cook on high pressure for 15 minutes.

2. Let the pressure release naturally for 10 minutes, then quick-release the remaining pressure. Plate the chicken. Spoon a little more sauce over the chicken and serve.

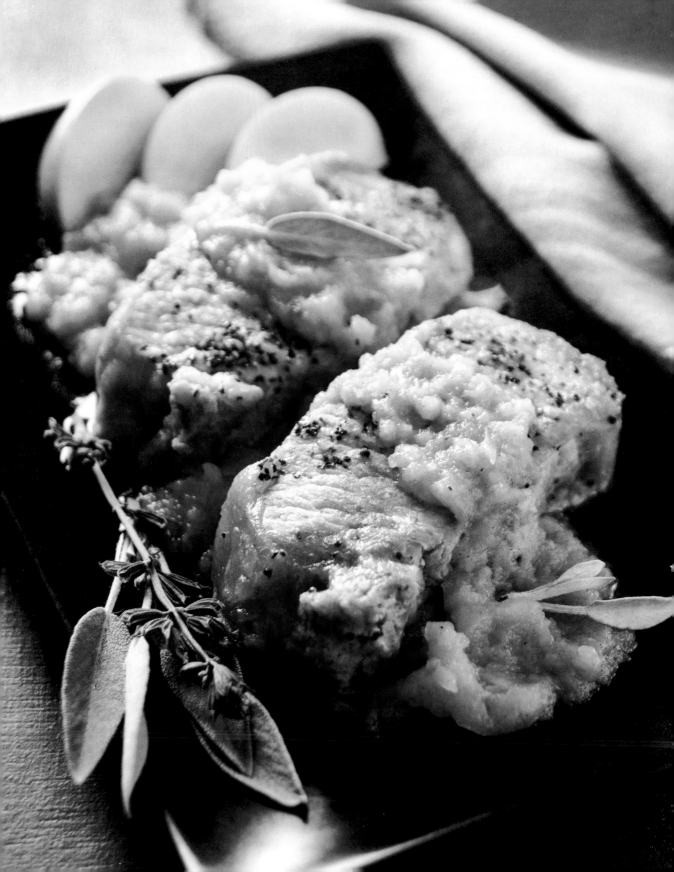

Cinnamon-Apple Pork Chops

These pork chops are a fantastic way to take advantage of fall flavors. If you don't have pumpkin pie spice, you can substitute ½ teaspoon ground cinnamon, ¼ teaspoon ground nutmeg, and ¼ teaspoon ground ginger. Or, you can just skip the spice mixture and add a second cinnamon stick.

Makes 2 servings | Serving size: 1 pork chop and ¼ cup apples | Cook time: 45 minutes |
Prep time: 5 minutes
Per serving: calories 377; fat 9 g; saturated fat 2.5 g; fiber 5 g; protein 42 g;
carbohydrates 30 g; sugar 22 g

1 teaspoon olive oil
2 (1-inch-thick) boneless pork chops
Kosher salt and freshly ground black pepper
2 Granny Smith apples, sliced
1 cinnamon stick
2 sage leaves, minced
1 teaspoon pumpkin pie spice
½ cup unsweetened applesauce
½ cup water

1. Set the Instant Pot to "sauté, medium heat." Once it reads "hot," add the oil and pork chops, sprinkle lightly with salt and pepper, and brown for 5 minutes, turning them over halfway through.

2. Transfer the pork chops to a plate. Add the apples, cinnamon stick, sage, pumpkin pie spice, applesauce, and water to the pot. Mix to combine and return the pork chops to the pot.

3. Cover and cook on high pressure for 10 minutes. Let the pressure release naturally for 10 minutes, then quick-release the remaining pressure.

4. Remove the pork chops and half the apples to a plate to rest. Set the pot to "sauté, medium heat" and cook to boil down the sauce until thickened, about 10 minutes. Pour the sauce over the pork chops and apples and serve.

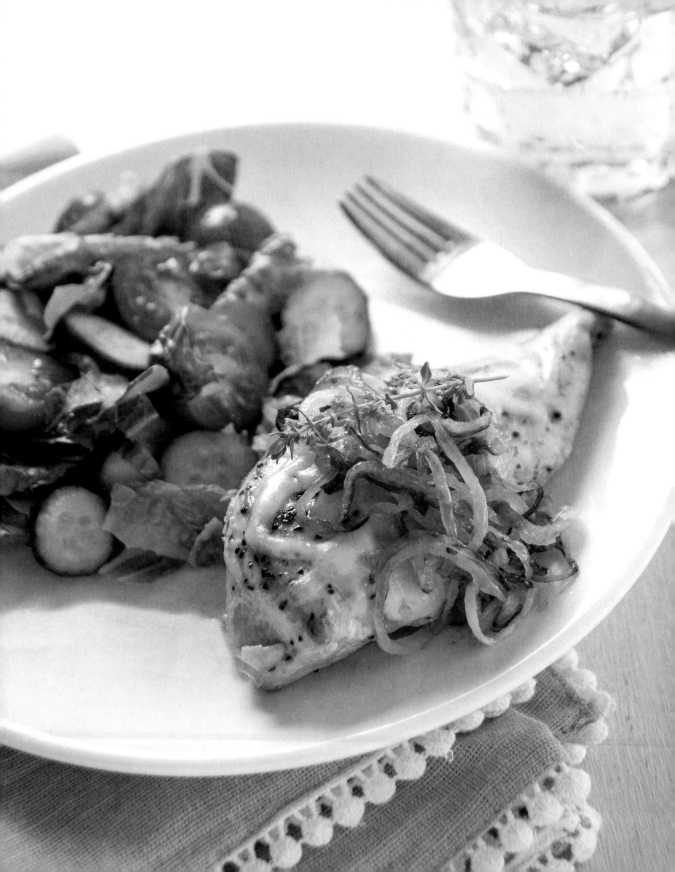

French Onion Chicken

This is one of my new favorite recipes, it's so easy and full of flavor!! I love to serve it alongside a salad or the Rosemary Fingerling Potatoes (page 77).

Makes 2 servings | Serving size: 1 chicken breast | Cook time: 45 minutes | Prep time: 5 minutes
Per serving: calories 419; fat 15.5 g; saturated fat 6 g; fiber 1 g; protein 61 g;
carbohydrates 6 g; sugar 2 g

---

1 teaspoon olive oil
1 yellow onion, halved and sliced thin
Kosher salt and freshly ground black
  pepper
1 fresh thyme sprig
2 garlic cloves, minced
1 teaspoon Worcestershire sauce
2 boneless, skinless chicken breasts
1 cup beef broth
⅓ cup shredded Gruyère cheese or 2 slices
  provolone cheese

1. Set the Instant Pot to "sauté, low heat." Once it reads "hot," add the olive oil, onion, a pinch each of salt and pepper, and the thyme. Mix to combine. With the pot loosely covered but not sealed, cook until the onion is sticky and golden, 10 to 15 minutes, stirring every couple of minutes.

2. Hit "cancel," then set to "sauté, medium heat." Add the garlic and Worcestershire sauce, mix to combine, and push the onion to the side of the pot. Add the chicken and brown for 2 minutes on each side (do all of this with the cover removed).

3. Add the broth. Cover and cook on high pressure for 10 minutes. Quick-release the pressure. Top the chicken with the cheese. As soon as the cheese melts, transfer the chicken to plates.

4. Set the pot to "sauté, medium heat," and sauté the sauce and onion for 5 minutes, uncovered. Remove and discard the thyme, then spoon the onion over the chicken breasts and serve.

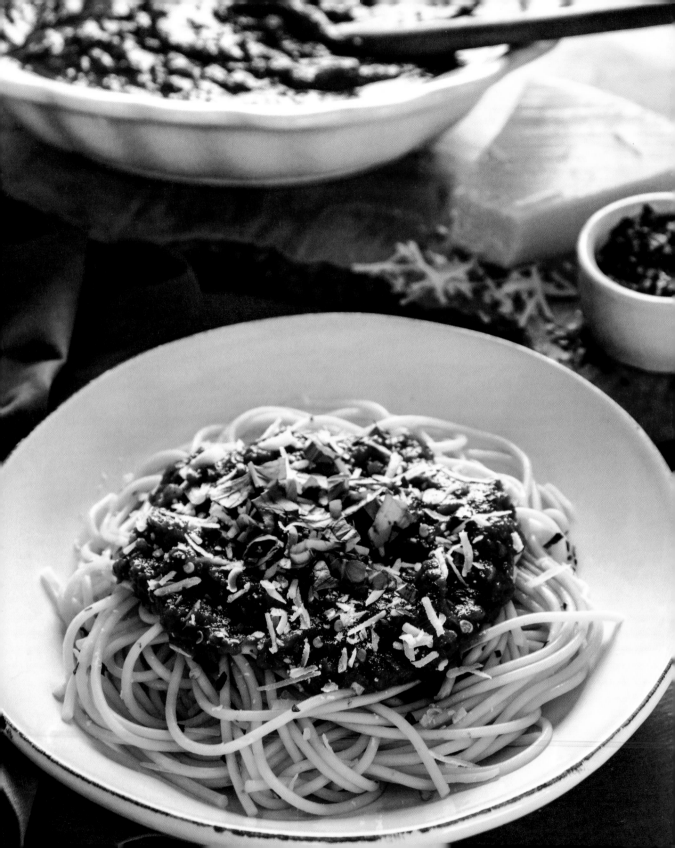

Fast Marinara

Confession: As an Italian woman I was very disturbed by the thought of cooking marinara sauce for just 30 minutes. I thought I might get struck down by lightning or become haunted by the ghosts of my Sicilian relatives! I even called my best friend, who married into an Italian family, and she agreed that it was just wrong . . . marinara should take a minimum of 4 hours, ideally 12 to 24 hours. But I gave Instant Pot marinara a shot, and I'm happy to report that it was excellent, with no hauntings or freak lightning strikes. I love this in the Italian Mac and Cheese (page 27).

Makes 8 servings | Serving size: ½ cup | Cook time: 45 minutes | Prep time: 5 minutes
Per serving: calories 103; fat 1 g; saturated fat 0 g; fiber 6 g; protein 3 g;
carbohydrates 20 g; sugar 12 g

---

1 teaspoon olive oil

1 yellow onion, minced

Kosher salt and freshly ground black pepper

4 garlic cloves, minced

¼ cup chopped fresh basil leaves (or 2 tablespoons Italian seasoning)

1 (28-ounce) can crushed tomatoes

1 (15-ounce) can tomato sauce

1 (6-ounce) can tomato paste

1 teaspoon sugar

1. In the Instant Pot, combine the olive oil and onion and sprinkle with a pinch of salt and pepper. Set the pot to "sauté, low heat," and cook for 3 minutes, until the onion starts to soften. Add the garlic and sauté for 2 minutes more.

2. Add the basil, crushed tomatoes, tomato sauce, tomato paste, and sugar. Cover and cook on high pressure for 25 minutes.

3. Let the pressure release naturally for 10 minutes, then quick-release the remaining pressure. Give it a good stir and serve over pasta.

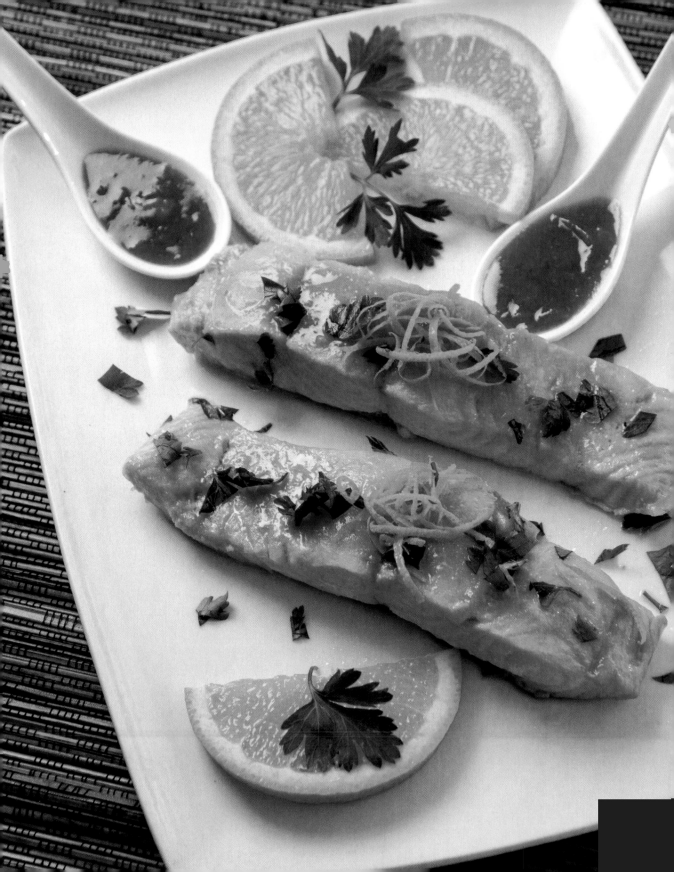

Orange Miso Salmon

I love miso and keep it in my fridge at all times. It adds wonderful flavor, but it can be difficult to find at the grocery store if you have never purchased it before. Look for it in the refrigerated section, often in the organic or all-natural section. And don't be shy about asking for help—I had to the first time. It lasts forever in the fridge, so don't worry about using it all right away. But if you want to skip it, just make marmalade salmon and it'll be delish.

Makes 2 servings | Serving size: 4 ounces | Cook time: 10 minutes | Prep time: 5 minutes
Per serving: calories 217; fat 10 g; saturated fat 2 g; fiber 1 g; protein 25 g;
carbohydrates 5 g; sugar 3 g

1 tablespoon miso paste

1 tablespoon orange marmalade

1 tablespoon soy sauce

1 cup water

1 (8-ounce) or 2 (4-ounce) salmon fillets

1. In a small bowl, combine the miso, orange marmalade, and soy sauce. Set the orange-miso sauce aside.

2. Pour the water into the Instant Pot and set the rack inside. Place the salmon on the rack, skin side down. Spread the orange-miso sauce over the salmon.

3. Cover and cook on high pressure for 3 minutes. Quick-release the pressure and serve hot.

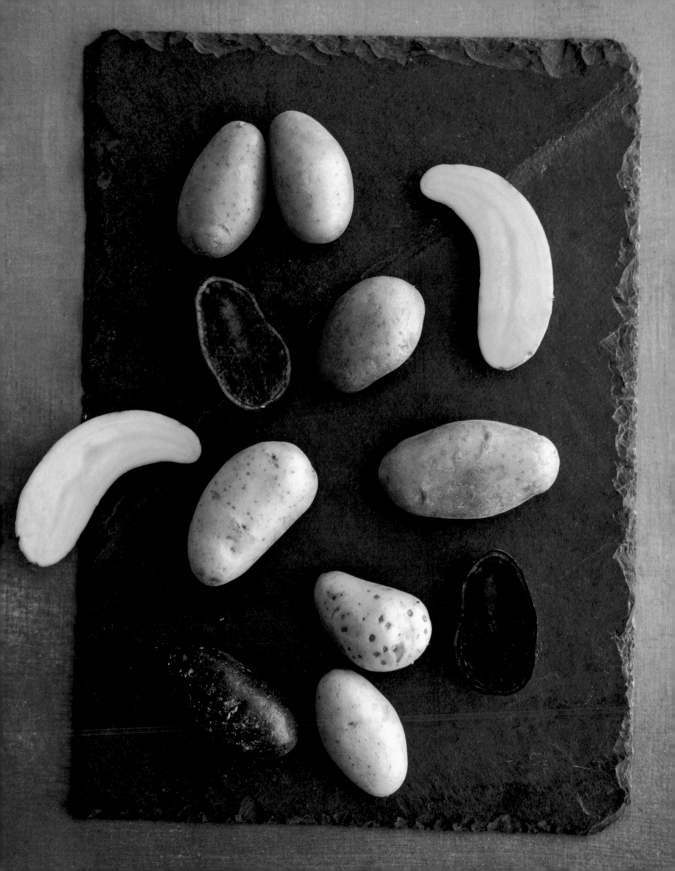

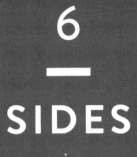

6
SIDES

These recipes go great with all your favorite main dishes. It's hard for me to pick a favorite, but I love the Bruschetta (page 69) on warm summer evenings and the Greek Rice "Bake" (page 73) with everything, anytime, including atop my favorite salads. And I could eat the Spicy Brussels Sprouts with Bacon (page 71) as a meal (every single day)! *Yum!*

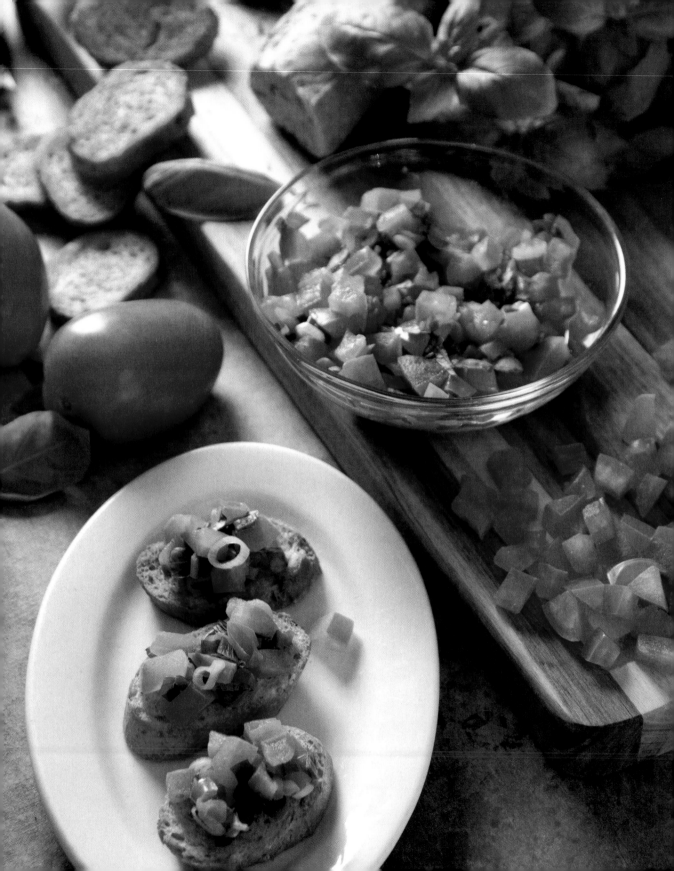

Bruschetta

I love bruschetta as a snack or appetizer; it also makes a great side dish with the "Rotisserie" Chicken (page 56).

This recipe calls for 4 slices of whole wheat bread, but if you're serving it at a party, get a baguette and slice it thinly for smaller, more elegant portions.

Makes 4 servings │ Serving size: 1 slice of bread and ¼ cup bruschetta topping │
Cook time: 15 minutes │ Prep time: 8 minutes
Per serving: calories 115; fat 1.5 g; saturated fat 0.5 g; fiber 4 g; protein 6 g;
carbohydrates 21 g; sugar 6 g

---

5 Roma (plum) tomatoes, cut into
　½-inch cubes
5 garlic cloves, 4 minced and 1 left whole
2 green onions, thinly sliced
½ cup water
4 slices whole wheat sourdough bread
½ cup chopped fresh basil leaves
Kosher salt and freshly ground black
　pepper

1. In the Instant Pot, combine the tomatoes, minced garlic, green onions, and water. Cover and cook on high pressure for 10 minutes.

2. Toast the bread, then rub one side with the whole garlic clove. Set aside.

3. Quick-release the pressure. Add the basil and a pinch each of salt and pepper and stir to combine. Spoon over the garlic-rubbed toast and serve.

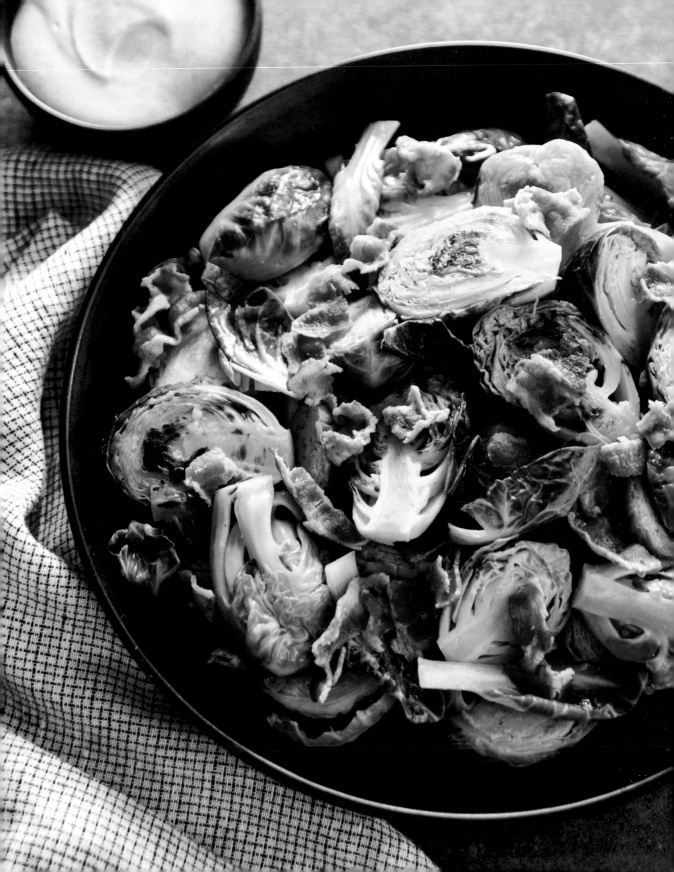

Spicy Brussels Sprouts with Bacon

Balance—that's what this recipe is all about. You can have your bacon and eat it, too, if you make it with a super-healthy veggie like Brussels sprouts! So yes, we are using *real* bacon. Go ahead and do a little dance; I'll wait here.

Makes 4 servings | Serving size: ½ cup | Cook time: 25 minutes | Prep time: 15 minutes
Per serving: calories 102; fat 5.5 g; saturated fat 0 g; fiber 4 g; protein 5 g;
carbohydrates 10 g; sugar 3 g

---

2 slices bacon, halved crosswise

1 pound Brussels sprouts, trimmed, dark outer leaves removed, halved through the stem

1 teaspoon smoked paprika

¼ teaspoon red pepper flakes

½ cup water

YOGURT TOPPING

¼ cup 0% Greek yogurt, store-bought or homemade (see page 19)

1 to 3 teaspoons sriracha, to taste

¼ teaspoon garlic salt

¼ teaspoon freshly ground black pepper

1. Line a plate with paper towels. Set the Instant Pot to "sauté, medium heat," add the bacon, and cook for 3 to 5 minutes, until crispy. Transfer to the prepared plate to drain. Leave the bacon grease in the pot.

2. Add the Brussels sprouts to the pot and sauté for 5 minutes, until lightly browned.

3. Meanwhile, in a bowl, mix the paprika, red pepper flakes, and water.

4. When the Brussels sprouts are finished browning, pour the paprika mixture over them. Cover, choose the "steam" setting, and cook for 4 minutes. Quick-release the pressure and drain the Brussels sprouts.

5. Meanwhile, make the yogurt topping: In a small bowl, combine the yogurt, sriracha, garlic salt, and pepper. Set aside.

6. Transfer the Brussels sprouts to a bowl, drizzle the yogurt topping over them, and crumble the bacon on top. Serve hot.

Skinny Creamed Corn

This creamed corn makes a great side dish for an easy weekday meal or a fancy holiday dinner. You can use whatever milk you have in the house, but I prefer unsweetened almond milk to keep the calories low.

Makes 4 servings | Serving size: ⅓ cup | Cook time: 20 minutes | Prep time: 3 minutes
Per serving: calories 190; fat 6.5 g; saturated fat 3.5 g; fiber 2 g; protein 6 g;
carbohydrates 27 g; sugar 8 g

---

1 (12-ounce) bag frozen corn kernels

1 cup unsweetened almond milk

3 tablespoons cream cheese

Kosher salt and freshly ground black pepper

1 tablespoon sugar

1. In the Instant Pot, combine the corn, almond milk, cream cheese, and salt and pepper to taste. Cover and cook on high pressure for 3 minutes. Quick-release the pressure.

2. Set the pot to "sauté, medium heat," add the sugar, and stir to combine. Cook until the sauce thickens, stirring often, about 5 minutes.

Greek Rice "Bake"

I made this rice to go with a roasted chicken and ended up adding it to everything I cooked for a full week. My favorite dish to add it to was salad. I made the Mediterranean Salad from my second cookbook, *Lose Weight by Eating: Detox Week*, added ¼ cup of this rice, and was in lunch heaven! Try this as a side dish or add it to your favorite salad all week for a hearty lunch. Or both! You'll save money if you use your leftovers wisely.

Makes 12 servings | Serving size: ¼ cup | Cook time: 20 minutes | Prep time: 10 minutes
Per serving: calories 104; fat 2.5 g; saturated fat 0.5 g; fiber 1 g; protein 7 g;
carbohydrates 13 g; sugar 0 g

---

1 teaspoon olive oil

½ red onion, minced

2 garlic cloves, minced

Kosher salt and freshly ground black pepper

1 cup brown rice

1¼ cups chicken broth or water

Grated zest and juice of ½ lemon

½ teaspoon ground cumin

1 tablespoon minced fresh dill or ½ tablespoon dried dill

½ cup chopped fresh spinach

2 tablespoons sliced Kalamata olives

1. Set the Instant Pot to "sauté, low heat." Once it reads "hot," add the olive oil, onion, garlic, and a pinch each of salt and pepper and sauté about 5 minutes, until the onion begins to soften. Add the rice and cook, stirring occasionally, for 3 minutes.

2. Add the broth, lemon zest, cumin, dill, and spinach. Cover and cook on high pressure (or the "rice" setting if there is one) for 3 minutes.

3. Let the pressure release naturally for 10 minutes, then quick-release the remaining pressure. Add the olives and lemon juice, mix to combine, and serve.

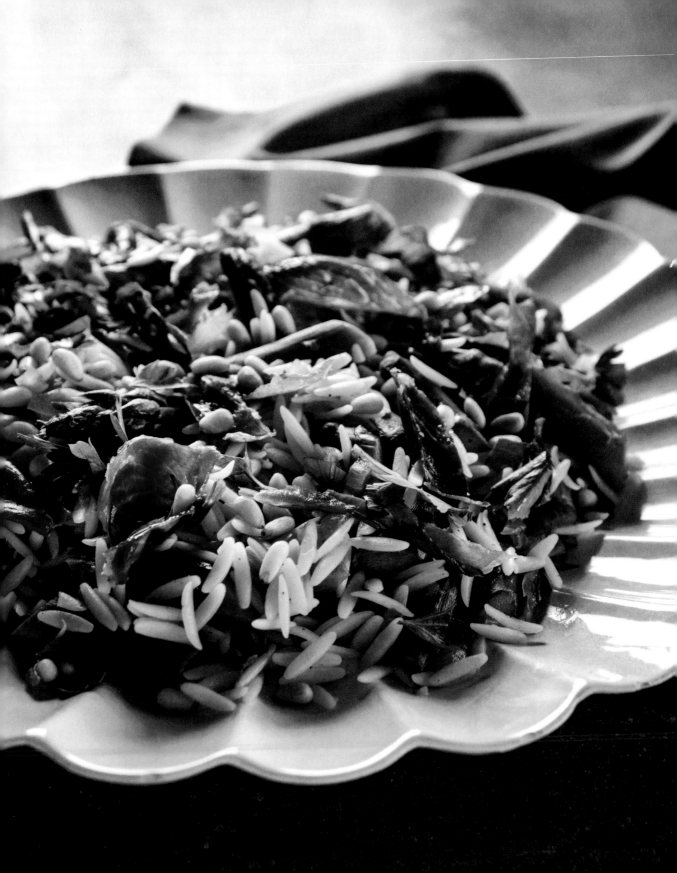

Asparagus and Orzo with Crispy Prosciutto

I try to be sure to use up any expensive ingredients throughout the week to stretch out my dollar. Not that prosciutto is all that expensive, but it's not cheap, either. So, if you've purchased prosciutto for another recipe, here's a great way to stretch your dollar and make an amazing side dish while you're at it.

Makes 4 servings | Serving size: ⅓ cup | Cook time: 25 minutes | Prep time: 5 minutes
Per serving: calories 61; fat 1.5 g; saturated fat 0 g; fiber 2 g; protein 4 g;
carbohydrates 9 g; sugar 2 g

½ teaspoon olive oil

2 slices prosciutto

1 bunch asparagus, trimmed and cut into ½-inch bites

1 yellow onion, minced

Kosher salt and freshly ground black pepper

½ cup uncooked orzo

1 cup water

2 tablespoons chopped fresh flat-leaf parsley

2 tablespoons pine nuts

1. Line a plate with paper towels. In the Instant Pot, combine the olive oil and prosciutto. Set the pot to "sauté, medium heat" and cook for about 5 minutes, until crispy. Transfer to the prepared plate to drain.

2. Add the asparagus and onion to the pot. Sprinkle with salt and pepper and sauté for 5 minutes, until the veggies start to soften.

3. Add the orzo and water to the pot. Cover and cook on high pressure for 3 minutes. Let the pressure release naturally for 10 minutes, then quick-release the remaining pressure.

4. Sprinkle with the parsley and pine nuts, then crumble the prosciutto over the top. Serve hot.

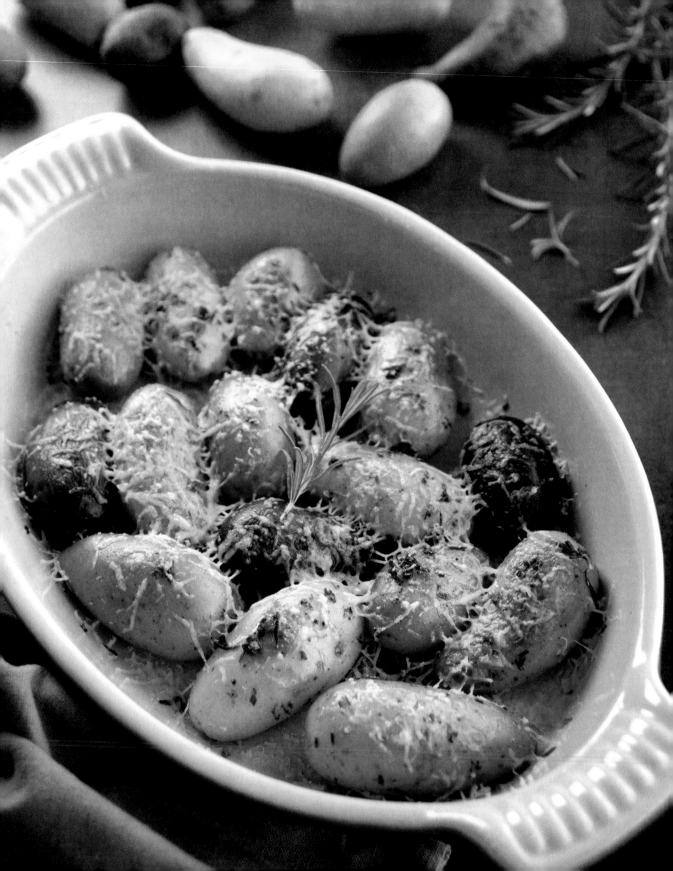

Rosemary Fingerling Potatoes

These are great alongside a roasted chicken or a nice steak. They're easy and flavorful, and make a terrific low-calorie side dish.

Makes 4 servings | Serving size: ½ cup | Cook time: 30 minutes | Prep time: 7 minutes
Per serving: calories 113; fat 2 g; saturated fat 0.5 g; fiber 3 g; protein 3 g;
carbohydrates 21 g; sugar 1 g

---

1 teaspoon olive oil

1 pound fingerling potatoes, washed

1 tablespoon chopped fresh rosemary

5 garlic cloves, minced

½ teaspoon kosher salt

½ teaspoon freshly ground black pepper

½ cup water

2 tablespoons grated Parmesan cheese

1. Set the Instant Pot to "sauté, high heat" and add the olive oil. While the olive oil heats up, poke the potatoes with a fork and drop them into the pot. Cook for 10 minutes, until lightly browned, stirring occasionally.

2. Add the rosemary, garlic, salt, pepper, and water. Cover and cook on high pressure for 7 minutes.

3. Let the pressure release naturally for 10 minutes, then quick-release the remaining pressure. Pour the potatoes and all the other contents of the pot into a strainer.

4. Preheat the broiler. Transfer the potatoes to a 9 × 13-inch baking dish. Top with any rosemary and garlic left in the strainer and the Parmesan and broil for 2 to 5 minutes, until golden brown.

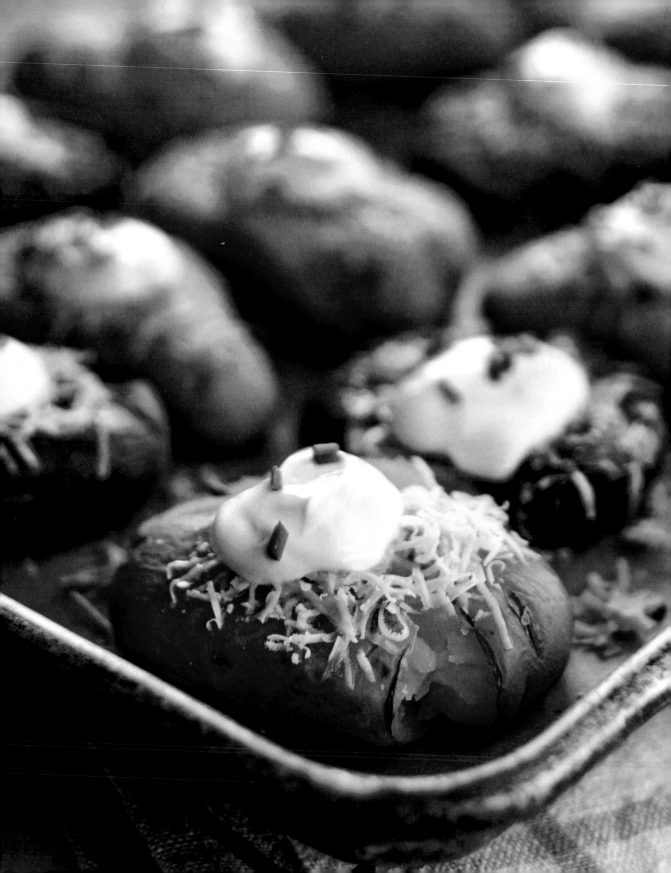

Herbed Smashed Potatoes

Smashed potatoes are so fun to make and eat, and so much easier with the help of an Instant Pot. These potatoes go great with a sprinkling of lemon zest on top or in the yogurt topping. You can swap out the rosemary for more thyme to cut costs, or swap out the Parmesan for cheddar cheese. It's a very versatile recipe, so get creative with the ingredients you have on hand!

Makes 4 servings | Serving size: 4 potatoes | Cook time: 30 minutes | Prep time: 10 minutes
Per serving: calories 63; fat 1 g; saturated fat 0.5 g; fiber 1 g; protein 3 g;
carbohydrates 11 g; sugar 1 g

---

1 small fresh rosemary sprig

3 garlic cloves, smashed

1 cup water

16 fingerling potatoes, washed

Kosher salt and freshly ground black pepper

1 teaspoon chopped fresh thyme

2 tablespoons grated Parmesan cheese

¼ cup 0% Greek yogurt

1 tablespoon minced fresh chives

1. Preheat the oven to 350°F.

2. In the Instant Pot, combine the rosemary, garlic, and water. Set the rack and steamer basket in the pot.

3. Prick the potatoes with a fork and place them in the steamer basket as you work. Sprinkle with salt and pepper and top with ½ teaspoon of the thyme. Cover and cook on high pressure for 10 minutes. Quick-release the pressure.

4. Carefully lift the steamer basket (use oven mitts) out of the pot. Transfer the potatoes to a baking sheet.

5. Use a spatula to gently smash the potatoes—just apply pressure with the back of the spatula until a potato starts to give. You want them still intact. Sprinkle with the Parmesan and some pepper.

6. Bake for 10 minutes, just until the cheese starts to melt.

7. Meanwhile, in a small bowl, combine the yogurt, the remaining ½ teaspoon of thyme, and the chives.

8. Remove the potatoes from the oven, add a dollop of yogurt topping to each one, and serve.

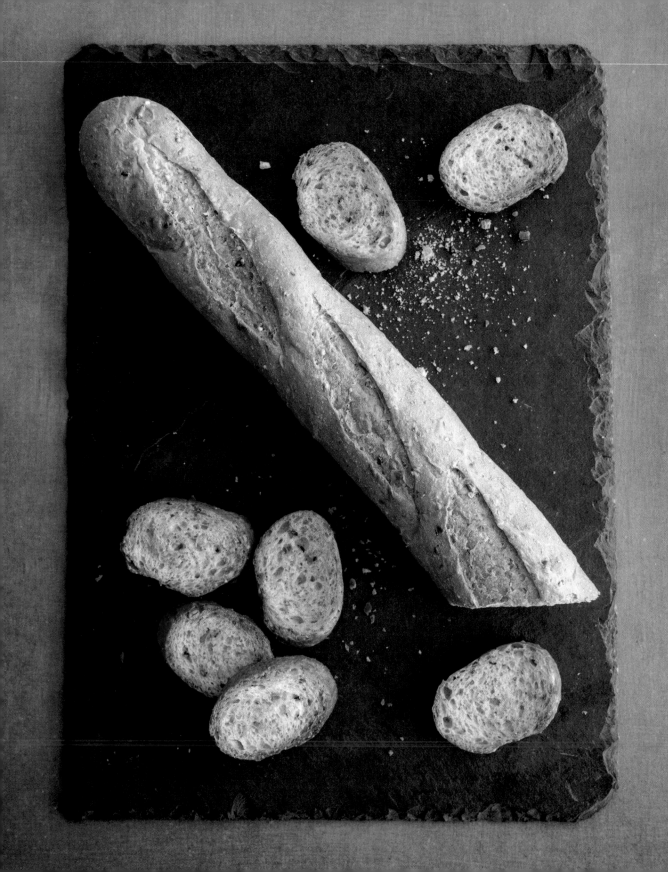

7
—
HOLIDAY FEASTS

Holidays can be so stressful, and unless you have two ovens (heck, even when you do!), there never seems to be enough room to get it all done. So why not make it easy on yourself and do a dish or two in your Instant Pot?! I love to cook the Scalloped Potatoes (page 91) and Spiced Carrots (page 92) the day before, move them to baking dishes, then reheat them the next day; this gives me the space in my Instant Pot to make the epic Green Beans with Bacon and Dates (page 87) or the Christmas Ham (page 85) on the day of the meal.

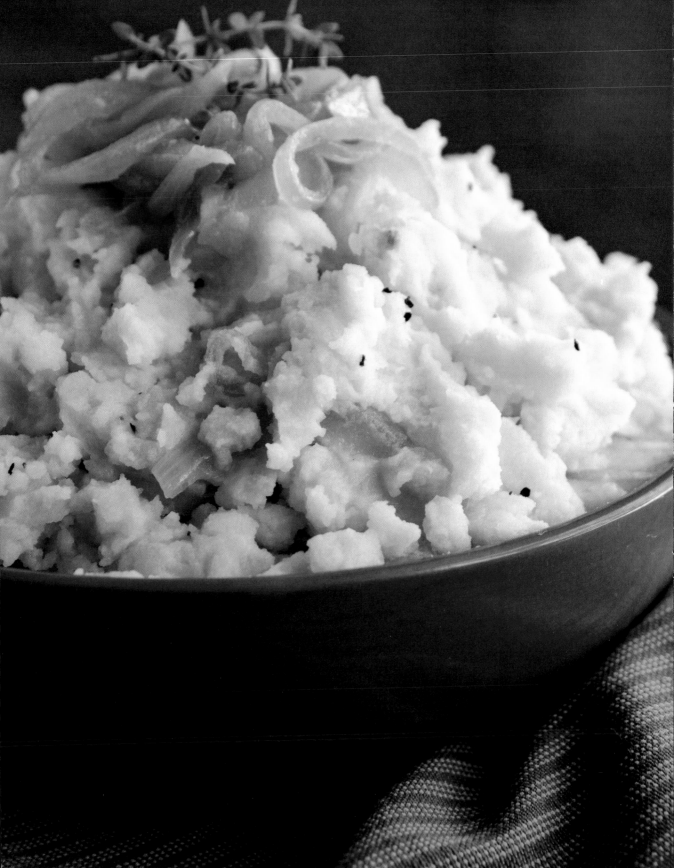

French Onion Mashed Potatoes

Mashed potatoes with a twist! You don't need butter and cream when you pack the recipe full of flavor.

I cut calories with smart swaps like using Greek yogurt and almond milk and by re-serving some of the potato water. Still want to add butter? Try using it on top instead, so that guests can indulge or abstain according to their preference.

Makes 10 servings | Serving size: ⅓ cup | Cook time: 45 minutes | Prep time: 15 minutes
Per serving: calories 158; fat 1 g; saturated fat 0 g; fiber 4 g; protein 4 g;
carbohydrates 34 g; sugar 4 g

---

3 cups water
8 large yellow-fleshed potatoes
1 teaspoon garlic salt
1 teaspoon olive oil
3 yellow onions, very thinly sliced
1 teaspoon fresh thyme leaves
2 teaspoons Worcestershire sauce
½ cup unsweetened almond milk
¼ cup 0% Greek yogurt
Kosher salt and freshly ground black pepper

1. Pour the water into the Instant Pot. Peel the potatoes and cut them into 1-inch cubes, dropping them into the pot as you work. Add ½ teaspoon of the garlic salt. Cover and cook on high pressure for 10 minutes.

2. Quick-release the pressure. Use a coffee mug to scoop out about 1 cup of the potato water. Drain the potatoes and transfer them to a large bowl.

3. Set the pot to "sauté, medium heat" and add the olive oil, onions, and remaining ½ teaspoon garlic salt. Cook for 10 minutes, loosely covered but not sealed, stirring often to avoid burning. Add the thyme and Worcestershire sauce, mix to combine, and cook for 3 minutes.

4. Add the almond milk and Greek yogurt and hit "cancel." Add the potatoes and use a potato masher to mash until smooth, adding the reserved potato water ¼ cup at a time to reach your desired consistency. Taste and add kosher salt and pepper as needed.

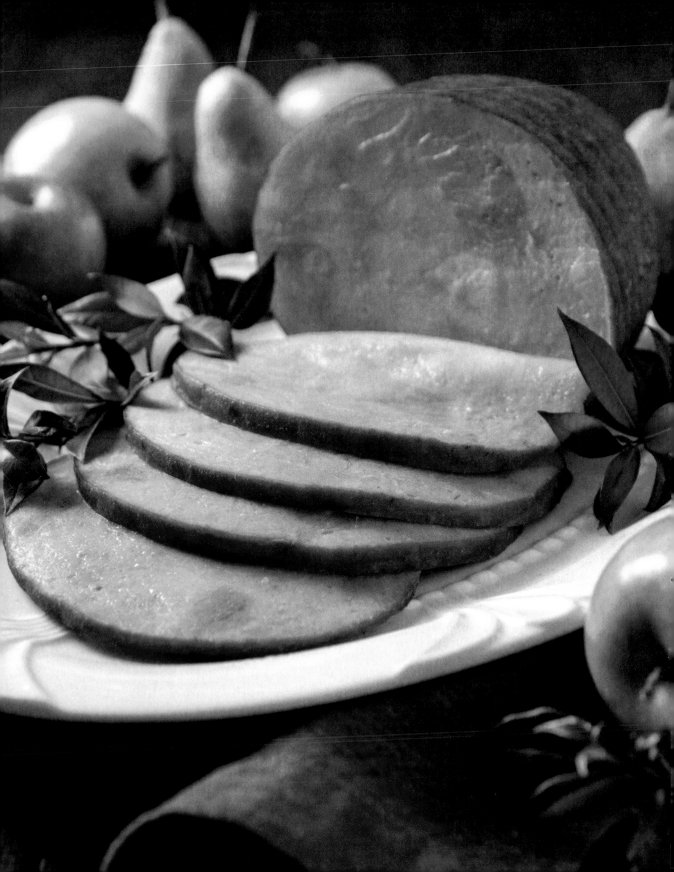

Christmas Ham

I like to use homemade Ginger Ale (page 119) in this recipe, but you can use a can of ginger ale, too. Of course, a bone-in ham is always preferable, but I find that most are too large to fit into an Instant Pot, so I call for the small "picnic" ham here.

Makes 10 servings | Serving size: 4 ounces | Cook time: 40 minutes | Prep time: 5 minutes
Per serving: calories 154; fat 5 g; saturated fat 1 g; fiber 0 g; protein 23 g;
carbohydrates 5 g; sugar 2 g

---

1 cup ginger ale, store-bought or homemade (page 119)
5 whole black peppercorns
1 (3-pound) boneless "picnic" ham
1 tablespoon honey
1 tablespoon Dijon mustard

1. In the Instant Pot, combine the ginger ale and peppercorns. Set the rack inside and set the ham on the rack.

2. In a small bowl, combine the honey and mustard. Spread it over the ham. Cover and cook on high pressure for 25 minutes.

3. Let the pressure release naturally. Remove the ham to a cutting board and let it rest for 15 minutes. Slice and serve hot.

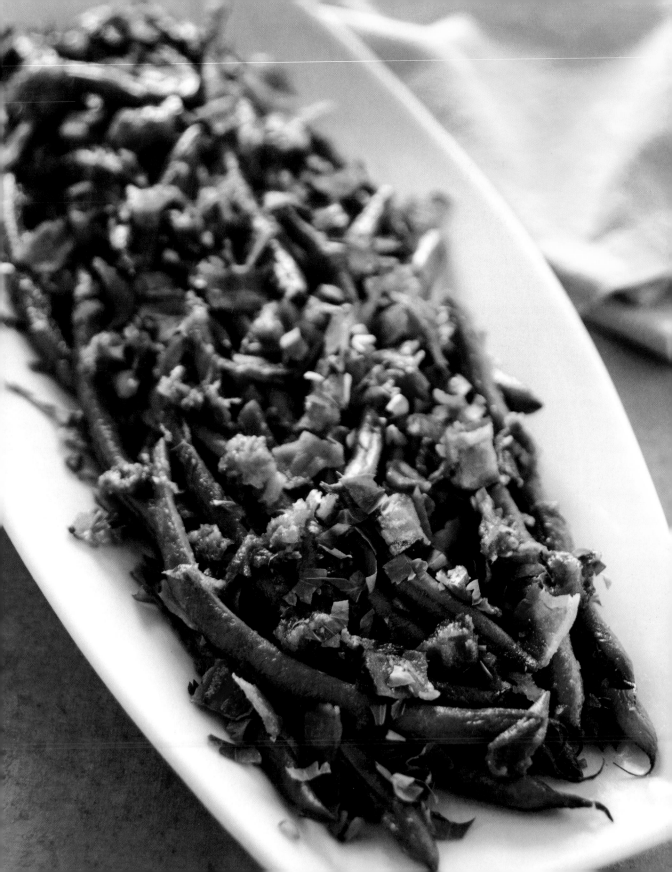

Green Beans with Bacon and Dates

I've never been much of a green bean fan, but I could eat these every day! Savory and sweet, soft and crunchy . . . perfect! They're a crowd-pleaser served with your holiday ham or roasted turkey.

The alcohol won't cook off here, but vegetable or chicken broth makes a fine substitute if you're serving this to kids.

Makes 4 servings | Serving size: ⅓ cup | Cook time: 20 minutes | Prep time: 10 minutes
Per serving: calories 106; fat 5.5 g; saturated fat 0 g; fiber 3 g; protein 3 g; carbohydrates 12 g; sugar 7 g

---

2 slices bacon, halved crosswise

1 pound green beans, trimmed

5 dates, pitted and roughly chopped

¾ cup white or rosé wine (or vegetable or chicken broth)

Kosher salt and freshly ground black pepper

1 tablespoon chopped fresh flat-leaf parsley (optional)

1. Line a plate with paper towels. Set the Instant Pot to "sauté, medium heat," add the bacon, and cook for 3 to 5 minutes, until crispy. Transfer to the prepared plate to drain, leaving the bacon grease in the pot.

2. Add the green beans to the pot and sauté for 3 minutes (this will help keep them firm).

3. Add the dates, wine, and salt and pepper to taste. Cover and cook on high pressure for 2 minutes. Quick-release the pressure. Drain the green beans and dates.

4. Transfer the green beans and dates to a serving dish and crumble the crispy bacon over the top. Sprinkle with parsley (if using) and serve.

"Roasted" Turkey Breast

I love making a turkey breast for small holiday gatherings, but that's not the only time I make it! I often pick up a turkey breast, cook it, and slice it thin for sandwiches and salads. I can't find a whole turkey year-round, but turkey breast is always available, so I take advantage of it.

Makes 10 servings | Serving size: 4 ounces | Cook time: 45 minutes | Prep time: 8 minutes
Per serving: calories 275; fat 12.5 g; saturated fat 3.5 g; fiber 0 g; protein 35 g;
carbohydrates 3 g; sugar 1 g

---

2 cups chicken broth

2 fresh rosemary sprigs

5 fresh sage leaves

5 garlic cloves, thinly sliced

1 orange, cut into ½-inch-thick slices

1 (2½-pound) bone-in turkey breast

1 teaspoon garlic salt

½ teaspoon freshly ground black pepper

1 tablespoon olive oil (optional)

1. In the Instant Pot, combine the chicken broth, rosemary, sage, garlic, and orange slices. Set the rack in the pot.

2. Sprinkle the turkey breast with the garlic salt and pepper and place it in the pot, skin side up. Cover and cook on high pressure for 25 minutes. Let the pressure release naturally to lock in the juices.

3. If you want the skin crispy, transfer the turkey breast to a roasting pan, rub it with olive oil, and place it under the broiler for 3 to 8 minutes. Watch closely so that it doesn't burn.

4. Let the turkey rest for 15 to 25 minutes before carving.

Cranberry Sauce

This recipe is great served hot, at room temperature, or cold out of the fridge. Make it easy for yourself and prep it a couple of days ahead; it holds beautifully in the fridge.

Makes 8 servings | Serving size: 2 tablespoons | Cook time: 30 minutes | Prep time: 3 minutes
Per serving: calories 89; fat 0 g; saturated fat 0 g; fiber 0 g; protein 0 g;
carbohydrates 22 g; sugar 20 g

---

4 cups fresh cranberries

1 cinnamon stick

3 dates, pitted and minced

½ cup water

2 tablespoons pure maple syrup

1. In the Instant Pot, combine the cranberries, cinnamon stick, dates, and water. Cover and cook on high pressure for 15 minutes.

2. Let the pressure release naturally for 10 minutes, then quick-release the remaining pressure. Stir in the maple syrup and serve.

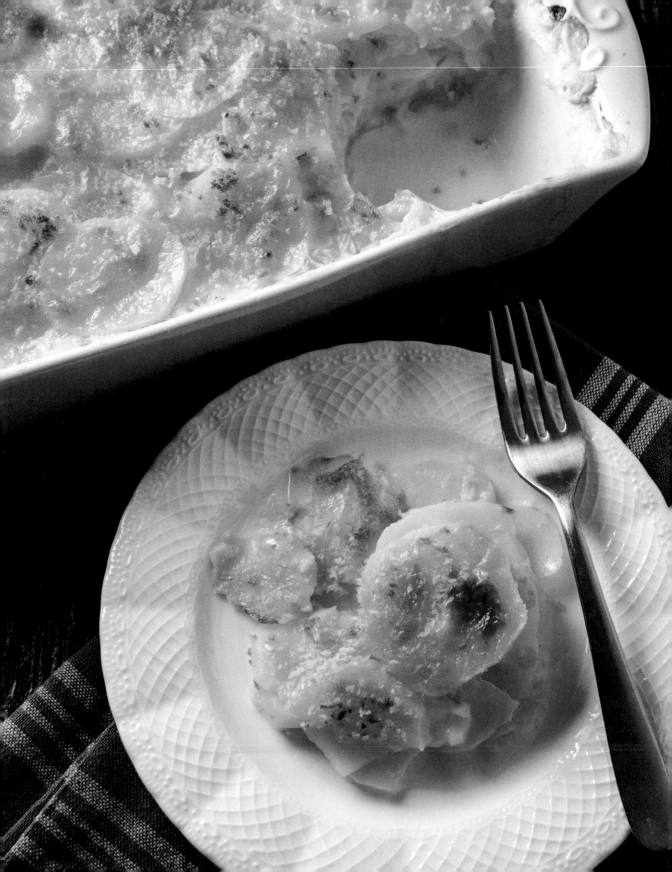

Scalloped Potatoes

Boxed scalloped potatoes are full of preservatives and chemical thickening ingredients that wreak havoc on your diet. Your body doesn't know how to process these fake ingredients, so skip the fake (and high-calorie) stuff and go all natural with this skinny version.

Makes 12 servings │ Serving size: ¼ cup │ Cook time: 25 minutes │ Prep time: 15 minutes
Per serving: calories 198; fat 6.5 g; saturated fat 3.5 g; fiber 3 g; protein 8 g;
carbohydrates 28 g; sugar 4 g

---

1 yellow onion, minced

2 garlic cloves, minced

1 teaspoon olive oil

Kosher salt and freshly ground black
    pepper

1½ cups 2% milk

8 Yukon Gold potatoes, peeled and cut into
    ⅛-inch-thick slices

¾ cup grated sharp cheddar cheese

3 tablespoons panko bread crumbs

1. Set the Instant Pot to "sauté, medium heat." Add the onion, garlic, olive oil, and a pinch each of salt and pepper and sauté for 5 minutes, until the onion starts to soften.

2. Add the milk and set the rack and steamer basket in the pot. Place the potatoes in the steamer basket. Cover and cook on high pressure for 5 minutes. Preheat the broiler.

3. Quick-release the pressure. Carefully lift the steamer basket (use oven mitts) out of the pot. Spread the potatoes in a 9 × 13-inch baking dish.

4. Hit "cancel." Remove the rack from the pot and add ½ cup of the cheese to the milk. Stir together until the cheese melts, then pour the cheese sauce over the potatoes.

5. Sprinkle the remaining ¼ cup cheese and the panko over the top of the potatoes. Broil for 5 minutes and serve.

Spiced Carrots

Carrots are a holiday staple in my family, so I had to attempt them in the Instant Pot. They were so easy and yummy that I ate the entire batch!

I like using full-size rainbow carrots for this recipe, but if you want to make it easier on yourself (no peeling or cutting), baby carrots work fine.

Makes 6 servings | Serving size: ¾ cup | Cook time: 15 minutes | Prep time: 10 minutes
Per serving: calories 71; fat 0.5 g; saturated fat 0 g; fiber 5 g; protein 1 g;
carbohydrates 17 g; sugar 9 g

---

2 pounds carrots, cut into large
  chunks
1 cup apple cider, store-bought or
  homemade (page 117)
1 teaspoon chili powder
½ teaspoon kosher salt

1. In the Instant Pot, stir together the carrots, cider, chili powder, and salt. Cover and cook on high pressure for 4 minutes. Quick-release the pressure. Transfer the carrots to a bowl.

2. Set the pot to "sauté, medium heat" and simmer the sauce, stirring often to keep it from burning, for about 5 minutes, until thickened. Drizzle half of the sauce over the carrots (discard the extra sauce), toss together, and serve.

Keeping It Healthy at a Holiday Gathering

Staying on plan through the holidays can be difficult; here are some quick tips to help you stay on plan and still enjoy Grandma's famous gravy:

PLATE EQUATION

You can still enjoy your favorite dishes at holiday gatherings. Follow the 50 percent vegetables / 25 percent protein / 25 percent carbohydrates per plate equation.

VEGGIES: Half of your plate should be vegetables. We already know that many vegetable dishes at holiday gatherings are unhealthy and full of empty calories. Bring a dish from this chapter (I highly recommend the Green Beans with Bacon and Dates, page 87). Or fill half of your plate with salad—you'll keep the calories low and won't feel guilty about dessert.

PROTEIN: I adore turkey—like really, really love it! And guess what?! Most often it's the protein at a holiday gathering that is lowest in calories and highest in nutrition. Feel confident in putting a big slice of turkey or ham on your plate.

CARBOHYDRATES: Skip the rolls and go for the potatoes! More nutritious, and let's face it . . . they're yummier, too. If you need to bring a dish to your gathering, the Scalloped Potatoes on page 91 are low calorie and impressive.

APPETIZERS, DESSERT, AND DRINKS

I'd like to take this opportunity to quote the great Julia Child: "Everything in moderation, including moderation." No time does this ring truer than at holiday gatherings!

APPETIZERS: Fill up on the veggie tray and pick one splurge. Does someone always bring the best mini quiches, or a dip that's to die for? Have a little—it's a party after all.

DESSERT: Don't deprive yourself of that end-of-the-evening treat—just split it with someone! A couple of bites of pie or cake is usually enough to satisfy, and if you just ate an entire holiday meal, you should already be full.

DRINKS: Start and end with water. When you arrive at the party or gathering, get a glass of water, then have one (just one!) glass of wine or a cocktail. End the evening with more water; this will get all that food moving through your body and help you avoid a food hangover the next day.

My last tip: Don't take it home! Or maybe take home some turkey or ham . . . but skip the leftovers and you'll be skipping hundreds of extra calories.

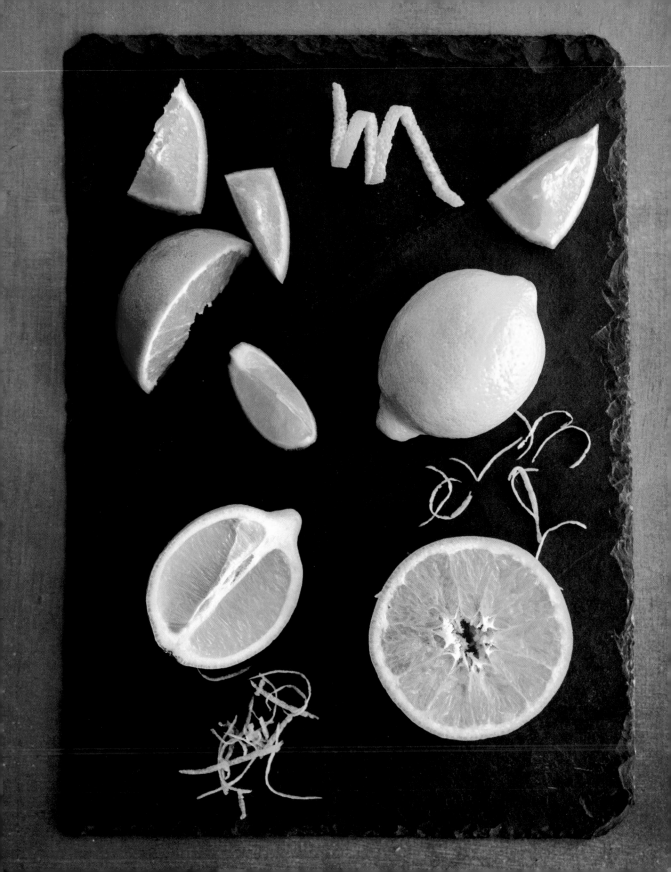

8
——

SHRED IT YOUR WAY

This chapter is special, the valedictorian of the book if you will. When I first started using my Instant Pot I loved how I could cook a ton of protein at the beginning of the week and use it throughout the week for fast, easy meals. With that in mind, I created this "Shred It Your Way" chapter. I have included directions on how to cook three proteins—pork, chicken, and beef—and recipes to use them in, so you can toss a meal together in no time. But what I'm really excited about is that all the subrecipes work with *all* the proteins! Yes, I paired the proteins with certain dishes, but the Steak Nacho Tostadas (page 107) can be made with the shredded chicken or the pulled pork, the Pulled Pork Sandwiches (page 104) are equally delicious with shredded chicken, and so on. Get creative and shred it *your* way . . . mix and match and have some fun!

Shredded Beef, see page 105

Shredded Chicken, see page 97

Pulled Pork, see page 101

Shredded Chicken

Shredded chicken in a flash! Need I say more? I add green chilies to give it an extra bit of flavor, but don't worry, it won't be too spicy. You can also add lemon juice and/or a chopped onion, or use vegetable or chicken broth in place of the water. It's versatile and easy.

Try this in the Chicken Salad Pitas (page 100) and the Chicken Club Wraps (page 99).

Makes 6 servings | Serving size: ½ cup | Cook time: 30 minutes | Prep time: 3 minutes
Per serving: calories 142; fat 3 g; saturated fat 1 g; fiber 0 g; protein 29 g;
carbohydrates 0 g; sugar 0 g

---

3 boneless, skinless chicken breasts

2 garlic cloves, smashed

1 teaspoon kosher salt

1 teaspoon freshly ground black pepper

2 tablespoons canned diced green
   chilies

1 cup water

1. In the Instant Pot, combine the chicken, garlic, salt, pepper, chilies, and water. Cover and cook on high pressure for 20 minutes.

2. Quick-release the pressure. Transfer the chicken to a plate and shred it to use as desired, adding ¼ cup of the cooking liquid to the chicken to keep it moist.

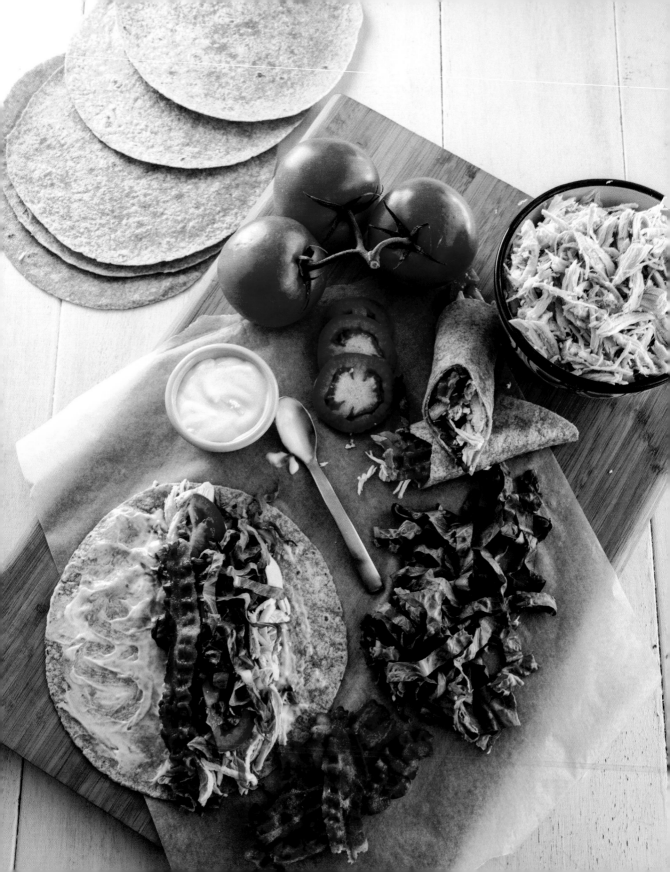

Chicken Club Wraps

Here's a great way to use the Shredded Chicken (page 97) for a quick lunch. These wraps travel well . . . and hold the phone, they call for real bacon! I know, right? Sounds too good to be true. You can use turkey bacon if you prefer, but it's just one slice and adds such a perfect crunch and flavor to this dish. Plus, it's a treat to be able to eat bacon and lose weight! It's all about moderation, and making a little of a yummy ingredient go a long way.

Makes 2 servings | Serving size: 1 wrap | Cook time: 15 minutes | Prep time: 7 minutes
Per serving: calories 322; fat 17 g; saturated fat 3 g; fiber 5 g; protein 20 g;
carbohydrates 22 g; sugar 4 g

---

2 slices bacon

⅓ cup 0% Greek yogurt

½ teaspoon garlic salt

¼ teaspoon Dijon mustard

2 (10-inch) burrito-size whole wheat
    tortillas

½ cup Shredded Chicken (page 97)

½ tomato, sliced

⅓ cup chopped romaine lettuce

1. Line a plate with paper towels. In a skillet, cook the bacon over medium-low heat until it's at your desired crunchiness level (very technical!). Transfer to the prepared plate to drain.

2. In a small bowl, mix together the Greek yogurt, garlic salt, and mustard.

3. Smear each tortilla with the Greek yogurt mixture and top with shredded chicken, tomato slices, romaine, and 1 bacon slice. Wrap them up like a burrito and enjoy now, or transfer them to parchment paper and take them on the road with you.

Chicken Salad Pitas

I love chicken salad, as you may already know if you have my other cookbooks. I think the chances of my cookbooks having a chicken salad recipe in them is about 95 percent, because I love it so much and because it's so versatile: you can get creative and never make it the same way twice. For this recipe, I tried some new ingredients, and I do think it's one of my best chicken salad creations . . . until next month, when I make it a new way.

Makes 2 servings | Serving size: 1 pita | Cook time: 0 minutes | Prep time: 8 minutes
Per serving: calories 242; fat 4 g; saturated fat 1 g; fiber 4 g; protein 29 g;
carbohydrates 24 g; sugar 7 g

---

1 cup Shredded Chicken (page 97)

¼ cup 0% Greek yogurt

1 tablespoon Dijon mustard

Garlic salt

1½ tablespoons minced shallot or red onion

10 red grapes, quartered

1 celery stalk, thinly sliced

Freshly ground black pepper

2 whole wheat pitas

½ cup baby spinach

1 tomato, thinly sliced

1. In a medium bowl, combine the chicken, Greek yogurt, mustard, ¼ teaspoon of the garlic salt, shallot, grapes, celery, and ⅛ teaspoon of the pepper. Taste and add more salt and pepper as needed.

2. Halve the pitas crosswise, then gently open them up, making 4 pockets. Divide the spinach among the pockets, top with tomato slices, and scoop ¼ cup chicken salad into each, spreading it out so that every bite gets some yummy chicken salad.

NOTE: If you're traveling with these pitas, wrap them in parchment paper or place them in travel containers. They travel well and make great picnic and lunch box meals.

Pulled Pork

This pork is incredibly versatile, and the Instant Pot makes it much faster than traditional pulled pork. I like to start the marinade as soon as I get home from the grocery store. If I know I'm going to make the pulled pork right away, I place the marinated pork in the fridge, but often I marinate the pork and freeze it so it's ready for me whenever I choose to make it.

Try this in Pulled Pork Tacos (page 103) or Pulled Pork Sandwiches (page 104).

Makes 18 servings | Serving size: ⅓ cup | Cook time: 1 hour 45 minutes, plus marinating time |
Prep time: 10 minutes

Per serving: calories 194; fat 9 g; saturated fat 3 g; fiber 0 g; protein 27 g;
carbohydrates 0 g; sugar 0 g

---

4 pounds pork loin, quartered
1 jalapeño, seeds and ribs removed
4 garlic cloves
Juice of 2 limes
1 teaspoon kosher salt
½ teaspoon freshly ground black pepper
1 cup water

1. Place the pork in a gallon freezer bag.

2. In a blender, combine the jalapeño, garlic, lime juice, salt, pepper, and water and puree until smooth. Pour the marinade over the pork and refrigerate for 2 to 24 hours.

3. Set the Instant Pot to "sauté, medium heat." Once it reads "hot," working in batches, add the pork and brown, transferring it to a platter as you go. Return all the pork to the pot, along with any juices on the platter and the marinade from the bag.

4. Cover and cook on high pressure for 80 minutes. Let the pressure release naturally for 10 minutes, then quick-release the remaining pressure.

5. Transfer the pork to a plate and shred.

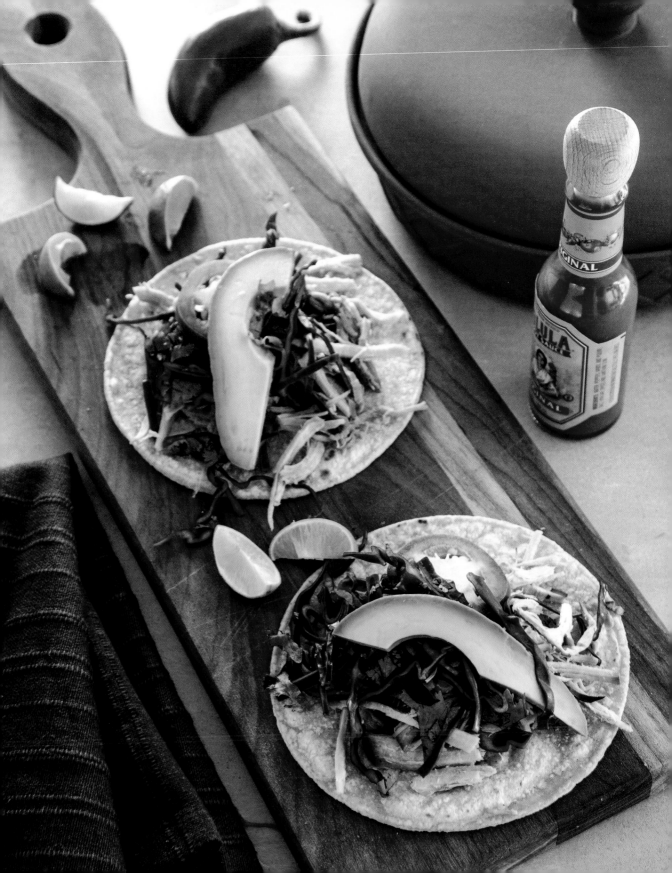

Pulled Pork Tacos

Taco Tuesday will never be the same after you make these yummy tacos! Just like all the recipes in this chapter, you can swap out the protein for your preferred protein. You can also make a taco bar with all three—the Pulled Pork (page 101), the Shredded Chicken (page 97), and the Shredded Beef (page 105).

Makes 4 servings │ Serving size: 2 tacos │ Cook time: 0 minutes │ Prep time: 10 minutes
Per serving: calories 268; fat 12 g; saturated fat 2 g; fiber 7 g; protein 16 g;
carbohydrates 27 g; sugar 2 g

---

1 cup shredded red cabbage

¼ cup chopped fresh cilantro

Juice of 1 lime

8 corn tortillas

1 cup Pulled Pork (page 101)

1 avocado, sliced into 8 slices

1 jalapeño, thinly sliced (optional)

Hot sauce (optional)

1. In a medium bowl, toss together the cabbage, cilantro, and lime juice.

2. To each tortilla, add 2 tablespoons pulled pork, some cabbage slaw, and a slice of avocado and dig in. If you like it spicy, add some jalapeño and/or your favorite hot sauce.

Pulled Pork Sandwiches

These sandwiches incorporate leftovers, saving you time and money. The leftover barbecue sauce from BBQ Chicken (page 57) is fantastic, but if you want to get some all-natural (organic is best) store-bought barbecue sauce, I won't hold it against you!

Makes 4 servings | Serving size: 1 sandwich | Cook time: 0 minutes | Prep time: 15 minutes
Per serving: calories 320; fat 5.5 g; saturated fat 1 g; fiber 8 g; protein 20 g;
carbohydrates 47 g; sugar 13 g

¼ red cabbage, thinly shredded
2 carrots, finely shredded
2 green onions, finely chopped
1 lime, halved
1 cup Pulled Pork (page 101)
¼ cup sauce for BBQ Chicken (page 57)
   or store-bought barbecue sauce
4 whole wheat burger buns

1. In a large bowl, combine the cabbage, carrots, and green onions. Squeeze half of the lime over the slaw and taste. Add more lime juice as desired.

2. In a medium bowl, combine the pulled pork and barbecue sauce, mixing well so that every bite is covered in yummy, sticky sauce.

3. Use your fingers to gently hollow out the tops and bottoms of the buns, to remove some carbs.

4. To assemble the sandwiches: Place ¼ cup of the pork mixture in each bottom bun half and top with slaw and the other half of each bun. Serve with lots and lots of napkins . . . this is a messy meal.

Shredded Beef

Here's another versatile shredded recipe. Any citrus can be used in place of the grape-fruit, so use what you have on hand. I love to prep this for the Beef Ragu Rigatoni (page 109); it's delicious and makes for a fast dinner that my kiddo never complains about.

Makes 8 servings | Serving size: ¼ cup | Cook time: 70 minutes, plus marinating time |
Prep time: 10 minutes

Per serving: calories 201; fat 8 g; saturated fat 3 g; fiber 0 g; protein 31 g;
carbohydrates 0 g; sugar 0 g

2½ pounds London broil steak, cut into quarters

1 yellow onion, sliced

4 garlic cloves, minced

1 tablespoon minced pickled jalapeños

½ cup fresh grapefruit juice

1 tablespoon chili powder

1 teaspoon ground cumin

Kosher salt and freshly ground black pepper

1 teaspoon olive oil

½ cup water

1. In a gallon freezer bag, combine the steak, onion, garlic, jalapeños, grapefruit juice, chili powder, cumin, and a pinch each of salt and pepper. Marinate for 2 to 24 hours in the refrigerator.

2. Set the Instant Pot to "sauté, medium heat." Once it reads "hot," add the olive oil and, working in batches, brown the steak, transferring it to a plate as you work.

3. Hit "cancel." Return the meat to the pot along with the water, the marinade, and any juices on the plate. Cover and cook on high pressure for 50 minutes.

4. Let the pressure release naturally for 10 minutes, then quick-release the remaining pressure.

5. Remove the meat to a plate and shred with two forks. Pour the liquid from the pot into a fat separator. Discard the fat and solids and pour ½ cup of the strained liquid over the meat and toss to keep it moist.

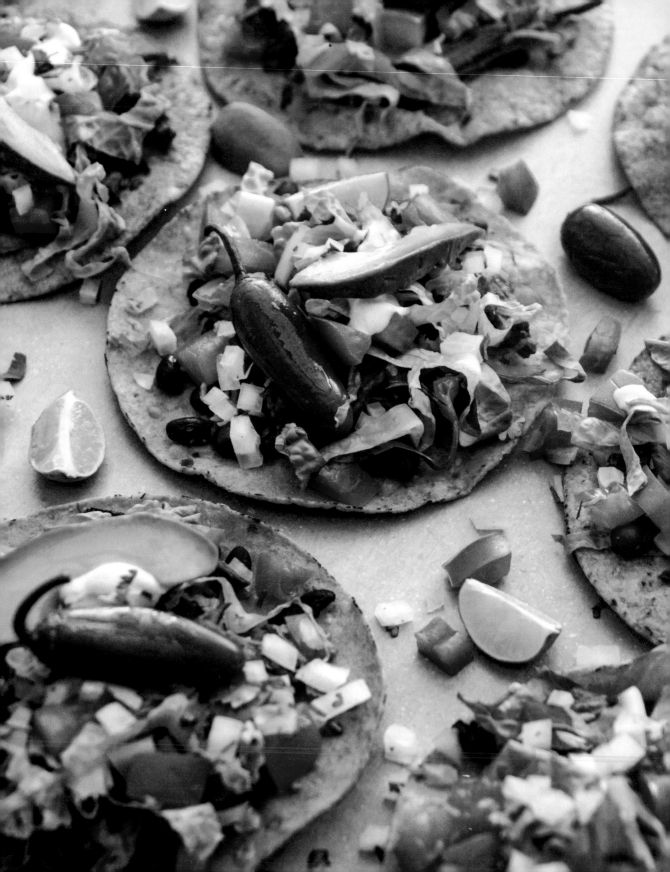

Steak Nacho Tostadas

I love these easy tostadas! They're like individual nachos—so fun. Feel free to pick and choose your toppings, but because we're trying to eat healthy, don't skip the veggies!

Makes 4 servings | Serving size: 2 tostadas | Cook time: 5 minutes | Prep time: 7 minutes
Per serving: calories 467; fat 19.5 g; saturated fat 8.5 g; fiber 12 g; protein 31 g;
carbohydrates 45 g; sugar 1 g

---

8 corn tostada shells
1 (16-ounce) can black beans, drained
   and rinsed
2 cups Shredded Beef (page 105)
1 cup shredded sharp cheddar cheese
2 cups shredded romaine lettuce
1 large tomato, roughly chopped

OPTIONAL TOPPINGS
1 avocado, thinly sliced
¼ cup Greek yogurt
Pickled jalapeños
Chopped onions
Hot sauce or salsa

1. Preheat the broiler.

2. Lay the tostada shells across 1 or 2 baking sheets. Top each with black beans, shredded beef, and cheese. Broil the tostadas for 2 to 5 minutes, until the cheese is melted.

3. Top each tostada with lettuce, tomato, and optional toppings of your choice (I love them all, especially Greek yogurt—it's just like sour cream!) and serve.

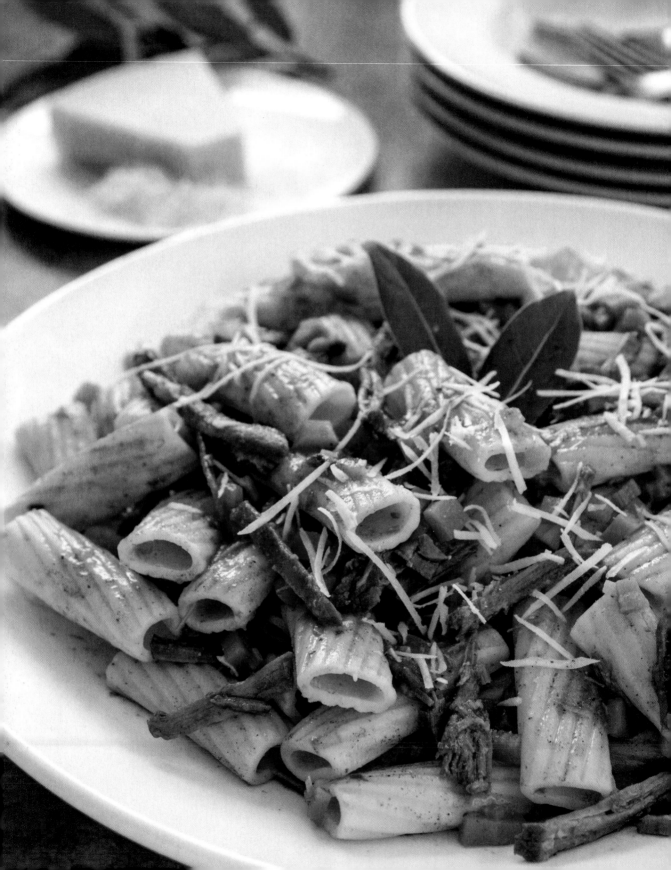

Beef Ragu Rigatoni

There is a restaurant here in town that makes amazing gnocchi and, yes, the potato pasta is wonderful; but what's really great about the dish is the beef ragu that tops it. The restaurant sells it for $14, and my daughter wants it every time . . . admittedly, so do I. That's $30 before tip—I can't afford that on a weekly basis! So, I had to re-create it at home, and this beef ragu is the perfect substitution. Best of all, I'm saving money *and* calories, cha-ching!

Makes 4 servings | Serving size: 1½ cups | Cook time: 20 minutes | Prep time: 10 minutes
Per serving: calories 208; fat 6 g; saturated fat 1.5 g; fiber 3 g; protein 18 g;
carbohydrates 21 g; sugar 4 g

---

1 teaspoon olive oil

1 yellow onion, minced

3 garlic cloves, minced

2 carrots, minced

2 celery stalks, minced

1½ cups beef broth

½ teaspoon minced fresh thyme

2 bay leaves

2 tablespoons tomato paste

Kosher salt and freshly ground black
   pepper

1 cup Shredded Beef (page 105)

8 ounces rigatoni pasta, cooked according
   to the package directions

Grated Parmesan cheese (optional)

1. Set the Instant Pot to "sauté, medium heat" and heat the olive oil. Add the onion and sauté for 5 minutes, until softened. Add the garlic, carrots, and celery. Sauté for 5 minutes, stirring often, until all the vegetables are softened.

2. Add the beef broth, thyme, bay leaves, tomato paste, and a pinch each of salt and pepper. Cover and cook on high pressure for 10 minutes.

3. Quick-release the pressure. Add the beef and set the pot to "sauté, medium heat." Simmer for 5 minutes, until the sauce has thickened. Add the cooked pasta and mix to combine.

4. Serve topped with grated Parmesan, if desired.

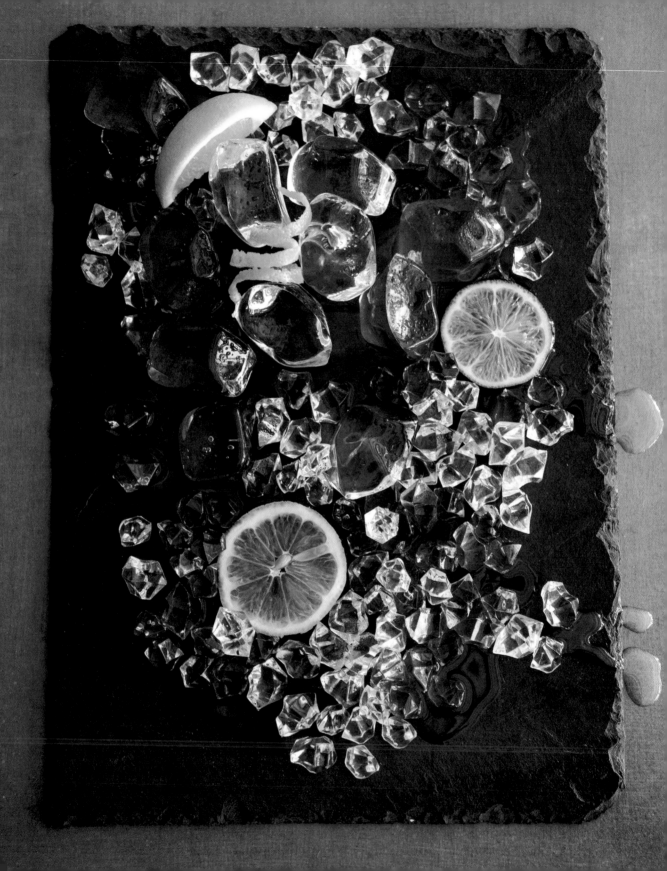

9

DRINKS

My first two cookbooks contained recipes for lots of fruit-infused water drinks, and I was planning on skipping the drinks chapter in this book . . . until I saw someone using the Instant Pot to make my infused-water recipes on the Internet. I was excited to try my own creations in a new way, but here I'm offering all-new flavor combos. You can use the Instant Pot to make the fruit-infused-water recipes in my other books, *Lose Weight by Eating* and *Lose Weight by Eating: Detox Week*; just follow the general directions in the recipes that follow.

Once I started on the fruit-infused waters I figured it would be easy to make iced tea (pages 113 and 115) and even homemade apple cider (page 117).

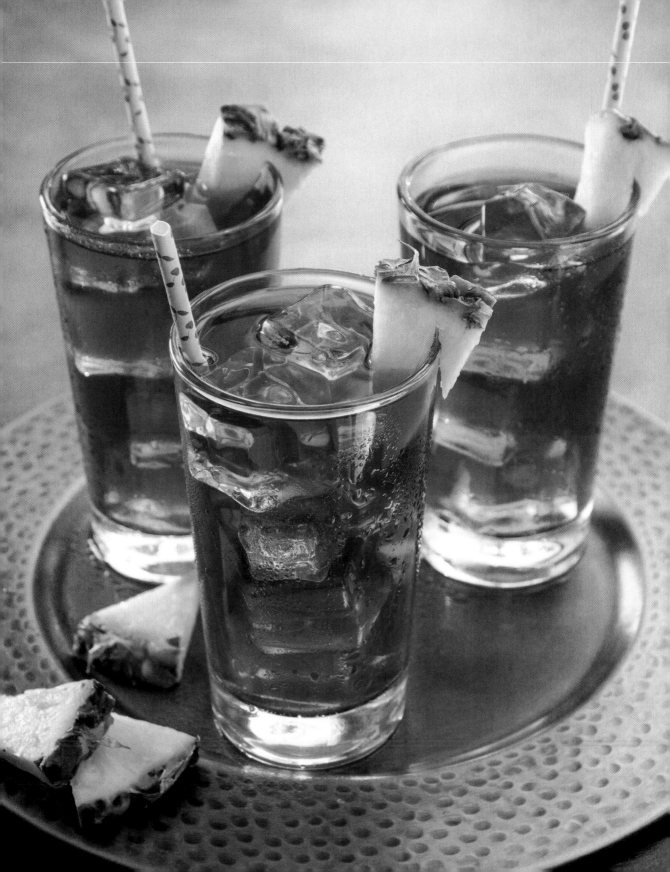

Pineapple Iced Black Tea

Oh . . . my . . . goodness! Have you had any of Starbucks's infused teas? They are amazing. Naturally I had to make a copycat (insert evil laugh here) so I can enjoy them at home anytime.

My favorite is the pineapple black tea, so I made it one spring afternoon and was instantly hooked! If you like a sweeter tea, add more fruit, and if you like a stronger tea, add an extra tea bag. This recipe is so easy, and you can make it at home for a fraction of the cost.

Makes 4 servings | Serving size: 1 cup | Cook time: 10 minutes | Prep time: 3 minutes
Per serving: calories 15; fat 0 g; saturated fat 0 g; fiber 0 g; protein 0 g;
carbohydrates 4 g; sugar 4 g

---

1 cup pineapple chunks (I use frozen)
2 black tea bags, outside wrapper removed
    and strings cut off
1 quart (32 fluid ounces) water

1. In the Instant Pot, combine the pineapple, tea bags, and water. Cover and cook on high pressure for 5 minutes. Quick-release the pressure.

2. Strain the tea (discard the solids), refrigerate until chilled, and serve over ice . . . or if you're like me and want to enjoy your "iced" tea as soon as it's done cooking (I have zero patience), just add a *lot* of ice to your cup and pour the hot tea over it.

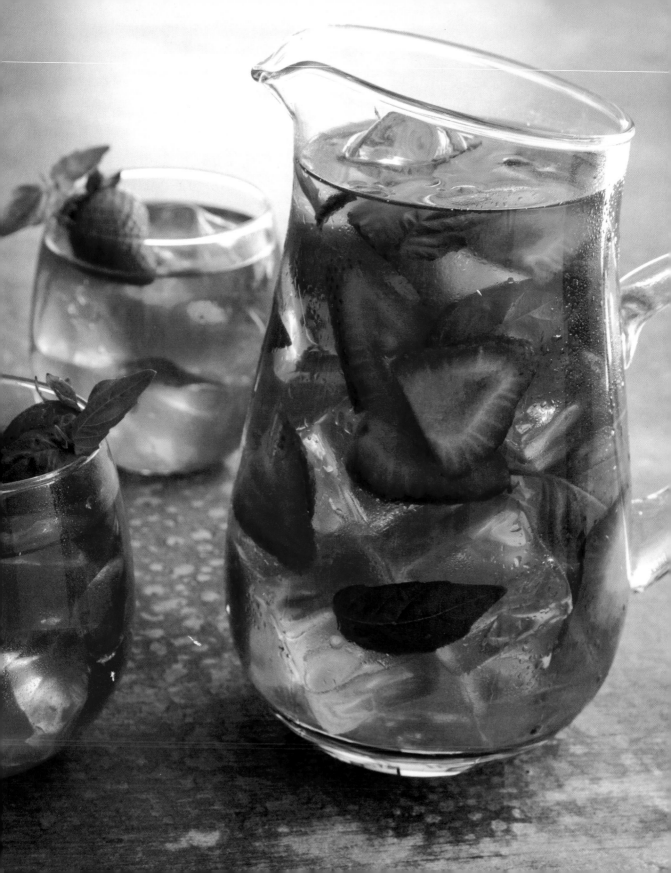

Strawberry-Basil Iced Green Tea

I love strawberries and basil together, and this recipe can be made as an iced tea or fruit-infused water (for an infused water, just omit the green tea bags).

Makes 4 servings | Serving size: 1 cup | Cook time: 10 minutes | Prep time: 2 minutes
Per serving: calories 9; fat 0 g; saturated fat 0 g; fiber 1 g; protein 0 g; carbohydrates 2 g; sugar 1 g

---

2 cups whole strawberries (I use frozen)

2 green tea bags, outside wrapper removed and strings cut off

1 quart (32 fluid ounces) water

2 fresh basil leaves

1. In the Instant Pot, combine the strawberries, tea bags, and water. Cover and cook on high pressure for 5 minutes. Quick-release the pressure. Stir in the basil and refrigerate the mixture until chilled.

2. Strain and serve over ice.

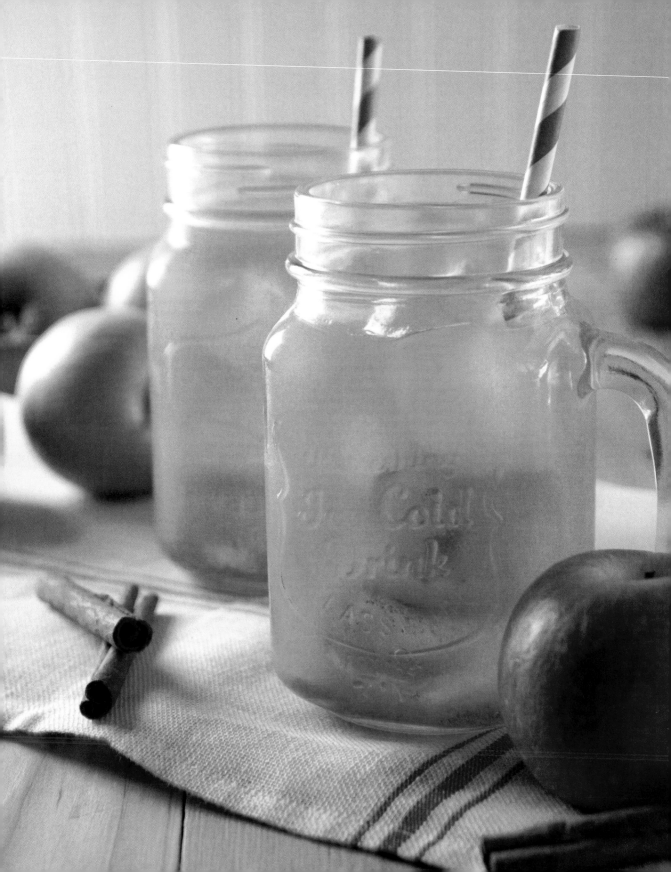

Easy Spiced Apple Cider

Who doesn't love apple cider? But those packets you can buy are full of preservatives and not at all healthy. This apple cider recipe is all natural *and* metabolism boosting— a drink you can splurge on without guilt!

Makes 4 servings │ Serving size: 1 cup │ Cook time: 30 minutes │ Prep time: 7 minutes
Per serving: calories 67; fat 0 g; saturated fat 0 g; fiber 2 g; protein 0 g;
carbohydrates 18 g; sugar 15 g

---

2 tangerines or 1 orange, peeled and segmented

3 Honeycrisp apples, cored and thinly sliced

½ tablespoon pumpkin pie spice

1 tablespoon dark brown sugar

1 quart (32 fluid ounces) water

1. In the Instant Pot, combine the tangerine segments, apples, pumpkin pie spice, brown sugar, and water. Cover and cook on high pressure for 15 minutes.

2. Let the pressure release naturally. Use a potato masher to mash up the fruit in the pot.

3. Strain the cider through a fine-mesh sieve (discard the solids). Serve the cider hot.

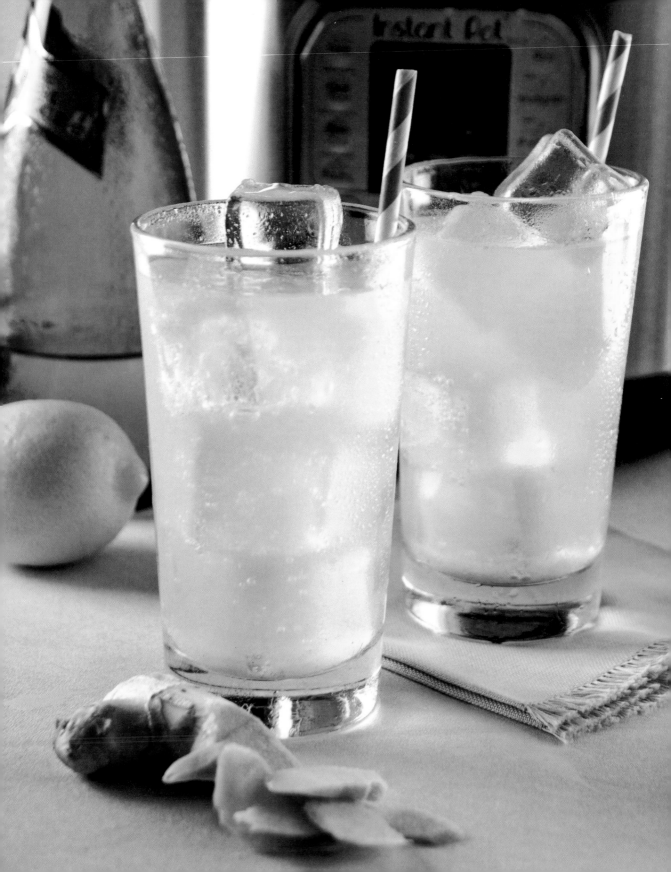

Ginger Ale

This ginger concentrate is delicious and easy to make, and if you have a soda maker in your house, as I do, you can use it to make all-natural ginger ale anytime you want.

If you don't plan on using the ginger concentrate all at once, just spoon it into an ice cube tray in 2-tablespoon portions, freeze, and transfer the cubes to a freezer bag. Pull them out one by one as needed!

Makes 10 servings │ Serving size: 1 cup │ Cook time: 40 minutes │ Prep time: 8 minutes
Per serving: calories 14; fat 0 g; saturated fat 0 g; fiber 0 g; protein 0 g;
carbohydrates 4 g; sugar 3 g

4-inch piece fresh ginger, peeled and cut
    into ¼-inch-thick slices
Juice of ½ lemon
1 cup water
¼ cup raw (turbinado) sugar
2 liters sparkling water

1. In a blender, combine the ginger, lemon juice, and water. Blend until smooth.

2. In the Instant Pot, combine the blended mixture and sugar. Cover and cook on high pressure for 30 minutes.

3. Let the pressure release naturally for 10 minutes, then quick-release the remaining pressure. Strain the liquid through a fine-mesh sieve (discard the ginger solids). Refrigerate the ginger concentrate until chilled.

4. For each serving, place 2 tablespoons of the ginger concentrate in an 8-ounce glass, add ice, and top up with sparkling water. Stir to combine and serve.

Blueberry–Apple Pie Infused Water

Try out my most popular recipe, Apple-Cinnamon Water, in a new way, with antioxidant-packed blueberries. I love how the blueberries give this drink some color. Most infused waters are very light in color, but add a few blueberries and you have a drink that looks as decadent as it tastes!

Makes 4 servings | Serving size: 1 cup | Cook time: 10 minutes | Prep time: 3 minutes

Per serving: calories 22; fat 0 g; saturated fat 0 g; fiber 1 g; protein 0 g;

carbohydrates 6 g; sugar 4 g

---

1 Honeycrisp apple, thinly sliced

1 cup blueberries (I use frozen)

1 teaspoon pumpkin pie spice

1 quart (32 fluid ounces) water

1. In the Instant Pot, combine the apple, blueberries, pumpkin pie spice, and water. Cover and cook on high pressure for 5 minutes. Quick-release the pressure.

2. Strain the water (discard the fruit) and refrigerate until chilled. Serve over ice. Will hold in the fridge for 3 days.

Berry Tropical Infused Water

I made this with blueberries, but I love that you can make this infused-water recipe with whatever berries you happen to have on hand. Strawberries work especially well, as do raspberries, but blueberries and blackberries will give this drink such a stunning light purple hue that you'll want to make it for all your parties.

Makes 4 servings | Serving size: 1 cup | Cook time: 10 minutes | Prep time: 2 minutes
Per serving: calories 27; fat 0 g; saturated fat 0 g; fiber 1 g; protein 0 g; carbohydrates 7 g; sugar 6 g

---

1 cup pineapple chunks (I use frozen)
1 cup blueberries (I use frozen)
1 cup mango chunks (I use frozen)
1 quart (32 fluid ounces) water

1. In the Instant Pot, combine the pineapple, blueberries, mango, and water. Cover and cook on high pressure for 5 minutes. Quick-release the pressure.

2. Strain the water (discard the fruit) and refrigerate until chilled. Serve over ice. Will hold in the fridge for 3 days.

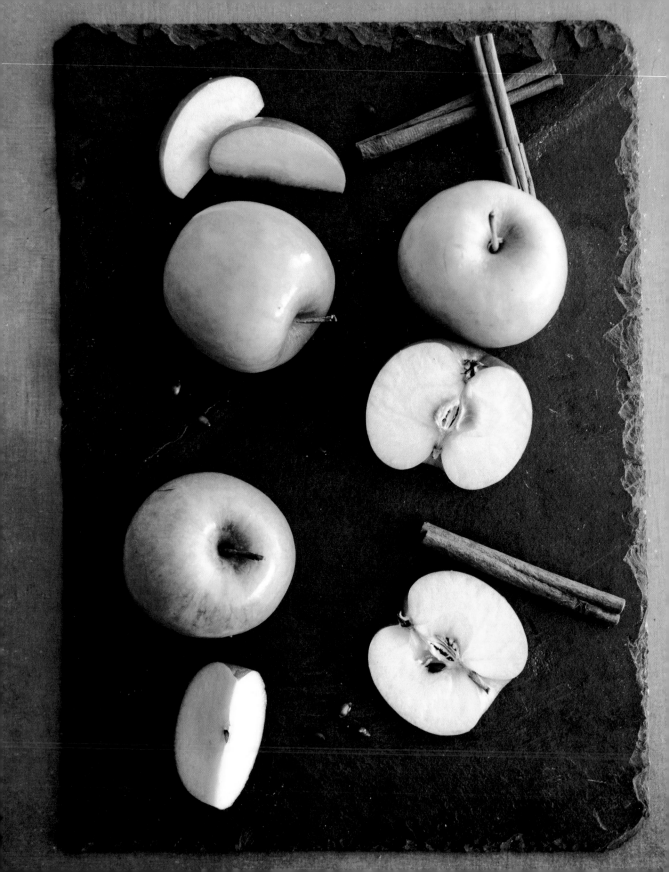

10

—

SWEETS AND TREATS

Usually the dessert chapter is my favorite chapter to work on when writing a book; I have a serious sweet tooth. But when it came time to test recipes for this chapter, I pouted like a child. I *love* to bake and wasn't thrilled at the idea of making bakery items in an Instant Pot.

Once I got started, though, I felt silly about my hesitation—baking Dark Chocolate Fudge Brownies (page 131) in an Instant Pot is life changing! You need to make them . . . like *now*!

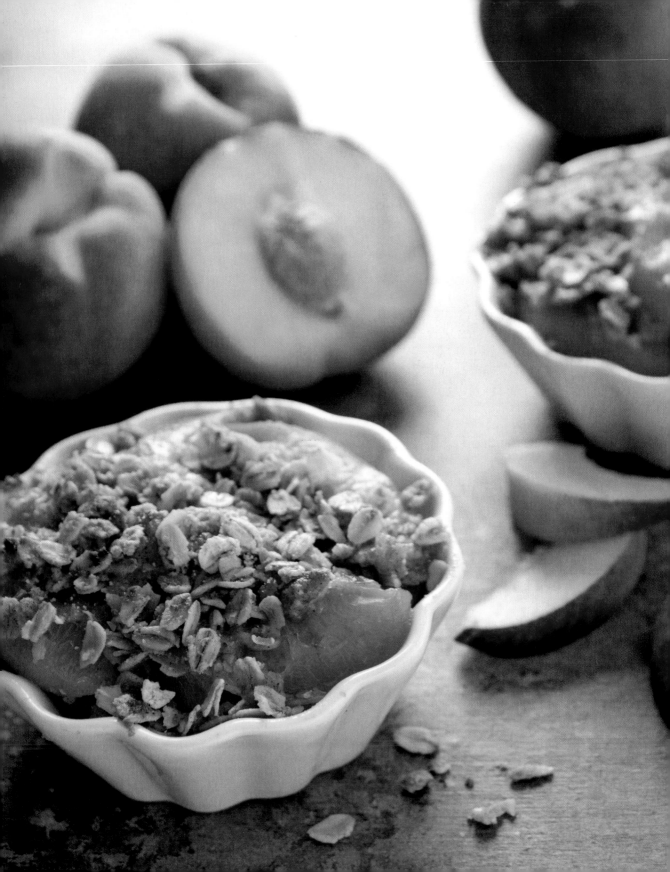

Ginger Peach Cobbler

These little individual cobblers are easy and satisfying, and they rely on peaches to sweeten the dessert, so you don't need so much sugar.

I like to use frozen peaches so I can skip the peeling and slicing—and it means you can make this yummy dessert in any season!

Makes 2 servings | Serving size: 1 ramekin | Cook time: 25 minutes | Prep time: 10 minutes
Per serving: calories 310; fat 4 g; saturated fat 1.5 g; fiber 7 g; protein 7 g;
carbohydrates 86 g; sugar 55 g

---

2 cups sliced peaches, fresh or unthawed frozen
1 teaspoon grated peeled fresh ginger
½ tablespoon dark brown sugar

TOPPING
½ cup old-fashioned rolled oats
¼ cup all-purpose flour
1 tablespoon dark brown sugar
1 teaspoon pumpkin pie spice

1 cup water
1 teaspoon unsalted butter

1. In a large bowl, combine the peaches, ginger, and brown sugar. Divide the mixture between two 6-ounce ramekins.

2. Make the topping: In the same bowl (for less cleanup!), mix the oats, flour, brown sugar, and pumpkin pie spice. Dividing evenly, sprinkle the topping over the peaches.

3. Pour the water into the Instant Pot and set the rack inside. Set the ramekins on the rack. Cover and cook on high pressure for 8 minutes. Quick-release the pressure. Carefully lift the ramekins (use oven mitts) out of the pot and transfer to a baking sheet.

4. Preheat the broiler. Drop ½ teaspoon butter on top of each cobbler and broil for 2 to 5 minutes, until nicely browned, keeping an eye on them to ensure they don't burn.

5. Let sit for 5 minutes before serving, so you don't burn your mouth . . . if you can control yourself.

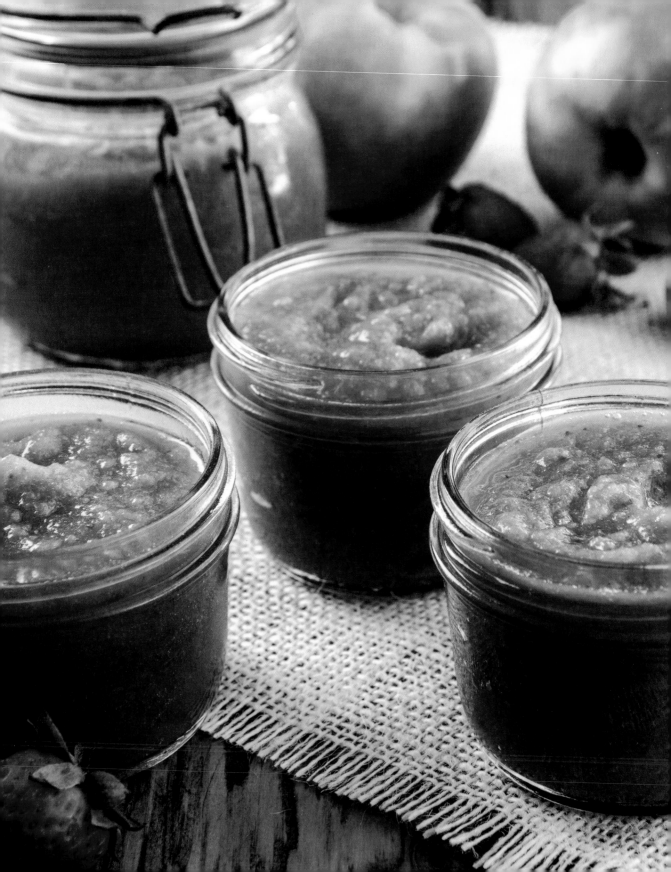

Strawberry Applesauce

You can get creative with this recipe! For cinnamon applesauce, use two more apples and two cinnamon sticks in place of the strawberries (just be sure to remove the cinnamon sticks before blending). For pear applesauce, use peeled and cored pears in place of the strawberries. Try any other berry, or mangoes, or even peaches!

Makes 6 servings | Serving size: ½ cup | Cook time: 20 minutes | Prep time: 10 minutes
Per serving: calories 94; fat 0.5 g; saturated fat 0 g; fiber 5 g; protein 1 g;
carbohydrates 25 g; sugar 18 g

---

5 Honeycrisp apples, peeled and cored
2 cups hulled fresh or frozen
    strawberries
½ cup water

1. Cut the apples into 1-inch chunks, dropping them into the Instant Pot as you work. Add the strawberries and water. Cover and cook on high pressure for 8 minutes.

2. Let the pressure release naturally (or it will spit all over your counter; trust me, I have made this mistake). Transfer the contents to a blender.

3. Blend, with the lid vented to avoid an applesauce explosion (wow, I'm making this sound like a very dangerous recipe). I like to remove the vent and cover it with a kitchen towel so the pressure from the hot sauce doesn't build up.

4. Transfer the strawberry applesauce to a large mason jar or small individual jars and refrigerate for 5 hours to chill completely. It will keep for 1 week in the fridge. (Alternatively, you can let the applesauce cool completely and freeze it flat in freezer bags. It will keep for up to 3 months.)

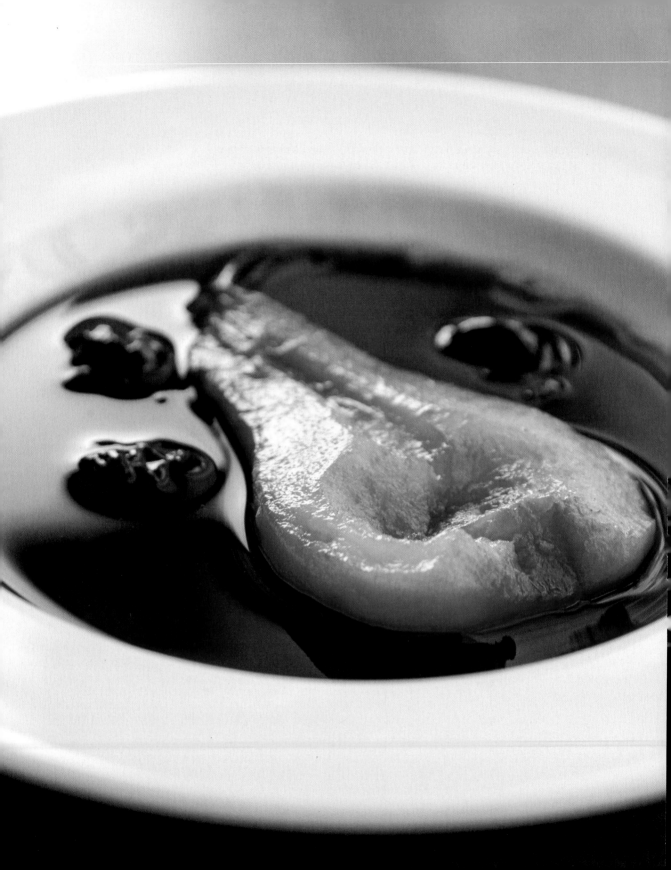

Rosé-Poached Pears

I don't know what's better, the delicious, complex flavor of these poached pears or the ombré color. They're perfectly pink on the outside, and when you cut into them the pink slowly bleeds to white. Simply stunning!

In this recipe the alcohol won't cook off completely, unlike poaching pears on the stovetop, so keep these as an adults-only treat.

Makes 4 servings | Serving size: ½ pear and 3 cherries | Cook time: 25 minutes |
Prep time: 8 minutes
Per serving: calories 88; fat 0 g; saturated fat 0 g; fiber 1 g; protein 1 g;
carbohydrates 22 g; sugar 21 g

2 cups rosé wine

½ cup raw (turbinado) sugar

2 cups water

2 pears, peeled, halved, and cored

12 pitted dark red cherries (I use frozen)

1 cinnamon stick

1 teaspoon pure vanilla extract

1. In the Instant Pot, combine the wine, sugar, and water. Set the pot to "sauté, medium heat" and simmer until the sugar dissolves.

2. Add the pears, cherries, cinnamon stick, and vanilla. Cover and cook on high pressure for 8 minutes. Let the pressure release naturally.

3. Transfer the pears and cherries to a large bowl. Remove and discard the cinnamon stick. Set the pot to "sauté, high heat" and simmer the remaining liquid for about 10 minutes, stirring to avoid burning. When it's syrupy, it's done.

4. Pour the syrup over the pears, cover, and refrigerate for at least 8 hours. Serve chilled or at room temperature.

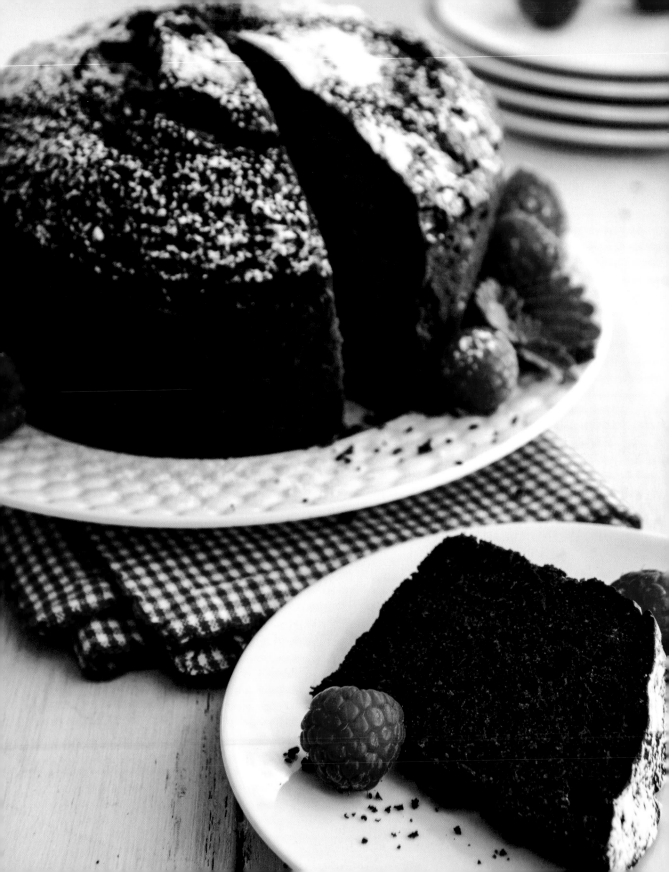

Dark Chocolate Fudge Brownies

I'm a brownie purist, so the thought of making brownies in an Instant Pot was disconcerting. However, I'm proud to say there have been brownie recipes in both my previous cookbooks, and that tradition was not about to end here, so I gave it a shot. To be honest, I complained for a full two days before testing this recipe. Well, talk about putting my foot in my mouth! They came out amazing, better than ever. So at least I had some yummy brownies in my mouth, as well as my size-eight foot. . . .

These brownies are perfectly chewy and never dry, thanks to the Instant Pot. So give them a try—if this brownie purist learned to love "baking" in an Instant Pot, so can you.

Makes 20 brownies | Serving size: 1 brownie | Cook time: 45 minutes | Prep time: 5 minutes

Per serving: calories 145; fat 8.5 g; saturated fat 5 g; fiber 2 g; protein 2 g; carbohydrates 16.5 g; sugar 7.5 g

---

¼ cup plus 1 teaspoon coconut oil

1 cup dark chocolate chips

½ cup sugar

1 cup 0% Greek yogurt

2 large eggs

1 teaspoon pure vanilla extract

½ cup unsweetened cocoa powder

1 teaspoon baking soda

1¼ cups all-purpose flour

½ teaspoon kosher salt

1 cup water

1. Place 1 teaspoon of the coconut oil in a 7-inch round deep ceramic dish and rub it around with your fingers to coat the dish completely. Make a foil sling (see page 5) and set it under the dish. Set aside.

2. In a large saucepan, combine the ¼ cup coconut oil, chocolate chips, and sugar and heat over medium heat, stirring until smooth. Set aside to cool to room temperature, 5 to 10 minutes.

3. Whisk in the yogurt, then whisk in the eggs and vanilla until combined. Whisk in the cocoa powder, baking soda, flour, and salt until you have a mousse-like batter.

4. Scrape the batter into the prepared dish and smooth it into an even layer. Pour the water into the Instant Pot and set the rack inside. Use the foil sling to lower the dish into the pot. Cover and cook on high pressure for 20 minutes.

5. Let the pressure release naturally for 10 minutes, then quick-release the remaining pressure. Carefully lift the dish out of the pot with the help of the sling. It will be hot—wear oven mitts! Place on a wire rack to cool for 20 minutes.

6. Use a knife to gently dislodge the brownies from the side of the dish, then place a plate over the top and flip the plate and the dish over. The brownies will slide out. Place another plate on top and flip again so that the brownies are right side up. Refrigerate for 20 minutes to chill, then slice into wedges, like a cake.

Stuffed "Baked" Apples

The beauty of the Instant Pot is that you can double or triple a recipe and the cooking time won't change because you're cooking under pressure. So it's easy to make this recipe with one apple or four. I can fit about six apples in my 6-quart Instant Pot.

I made this a "for each serving" recipe, because sometimes you just need to indulge in a snack for one. So, for each serving, here is what you will need:

Makes 1 serving | Serving size: 1 apple | Cook time: 10 minutes | Prep time: 8 minutes
Per serving: calories 120; fat 1 g; saturated fat 0 g; fiber 5 g; protein 1 g;
carbohydrates 27 g; sugar 19 g

---

1 teaspoon old-fashioned rolled oats
1 pecan, chopped
1 teaspoon chopped dried cranberries
¼ teaspoon pumpkin pie spice
½ teaspoon pure maple syrup
1 tablespoon plus 1 cup water
1 Granny Smith apple

1. In a small bowl, combine the oats, pecan, cranberries, pumpkin pie spice, maple syrup, and 1 tablespoon of the water.

2. Slice off the bottom ¼ inch of the apple so it will sit flat. At the stem end, use a paring knife to cut a ring around the stem and down around the core. Use a small spoon to remove the core and seeds, leaving a spot for the filling. Add the filling to the apple with a spoon, pressing down gently so it will all fit.

3. Pour the 1 cup water into the Instant Pot and set the rack inside. Place the apple stem side up on the rack. (Alternatively, you can place the apple in a ramekin.) Cover and cook on high pressure for 3 minutes.

4. Quick-release the pressure. Transfer the apple to a plate and remove the skin (it will fall right off) and discard. Serve the apple hot and bubbling.

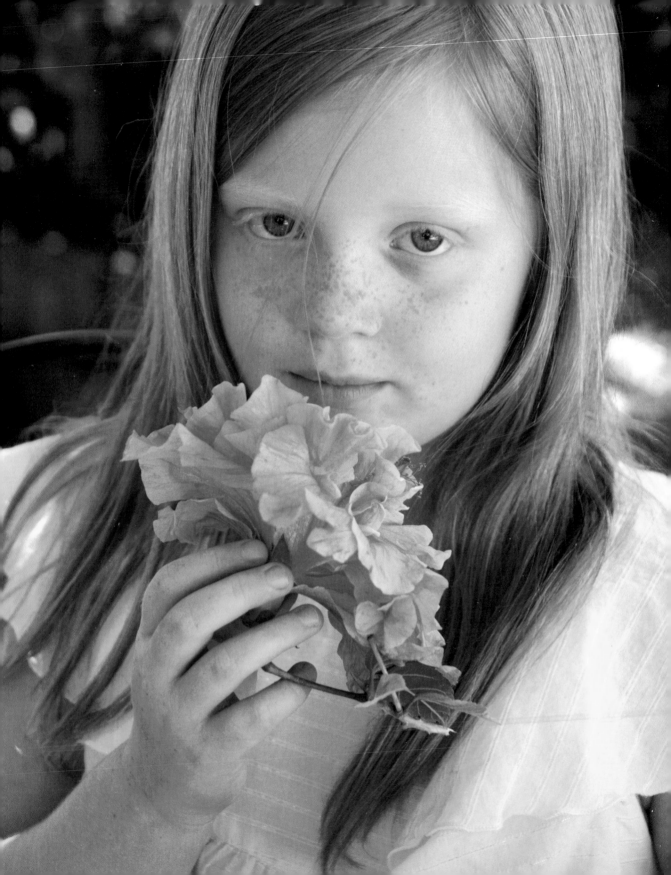

Acknowledgments

Thank you, Sophia, for being such a great kitchen helper while I tested these recipes and wrote this book. There is no greater joy than cooking with you, my sweet little girl!

Kara, thank you for being my rock! And for not ratting me out to the Italian Food Police for making marinara sauce in just 30 minutes.

Thank you, Sarah Passick, Anna Petkovich, and Celeste Fine, for being so supportive. Without you as my agents, this book never would have happened.

To Cassie Jones, Kara Zauberman, Heidi Richter, Andrew Gibeley, and everyone at William Morrow/HarperCollins, thank you for helping me make this book as beautiful as it can be, for fixing my multiple spelling mistakes, and for helping me make it a huge success.

To my amazing food stylist, Cindy Epstein. Over the years of working together we have become such fast friends—I adore you! I'm so blessed to call you my friend. Thank you for making my recipes look so scrumptious. To Carl Kravats, my incredible photographer, your work never ceases to amaze me. I'm so thrilled we have gotten to work on three books together! And of course, to the gal who makes it all possible, Joni, my chef and kitchen goddess, thank you for all you do to help put a book together.

To all my friends who helped me test recipes when you thought you were just getting a free meal . . . thank you, and I'm sorry. Special thanks to Scott, who never balked at my limited gluten-free cooking abilities, and was always so kind with recipe test notes.

To all my readers, thank you for buying my books, and for asking for more. Without you, my cookbooks wouldn't happen.

To my amazing aunt Laurie, who is one of my dearest friends, thank you for driving out and taking such great care of me after surgery so I could meet my editing deadlines. Your generosity surpasses your baking abilities, and that's saying a lot! Please send more peach cobbler and lemon bars . . . XO

To my dear friends Brian and Sue, thank you for being an amazing support system! I'm so lucky to know you both, and look forward to more years of friendship. I know, I know, I owe you both more brownies. . . .

Finally, to all the women I have met over the last year at Faces of Hope, Boise. You inspire me every day. You got out of unfortunate situations, and somehow you are stronger and more incredible each week. Thank you for holding my hand, for encouraging me, and for jumping to my side whenever I have asked.

Universal Conversion Chart

OVEN TEMPERATURE EQUIVALENTS

250°F = 120°C   350°F = 180°C   450°F = 230°C

275°F = 135°C   375°F = 190°C   475°F = 240°C

300°F = 150°C   400°F = 200°C   500°F = 260°C

325°F = 160°C   425°F = 220°C

MEASUREMENT EQUIVALENTS

Measurements should always be level unless directed otherwise.

⅛ teaspoon = 0.5 mL

¼ teaspoon = 1 mL

½ teaspoon = 2 mL

1 teaspoon = 5 mL

1 tablespoon = 3 teaspoons = ½ fluid ounce = 15 mL

2 tablespoons = ⅛ cup = 1 fluid ounce = 30 mL

4 tablespoons = ¼ cup = 2 fluid ounces = 60 mL

5⅓ tablespoons = ⅓ cup = 3 fluid ounces = 80 mL

8 tablespoons = ½ cup = 4 fluid ounces = 120 mL

10⅔ tablespoons = ⅔ cup = 5 fluid ounces = 160 mL

12 tablespoons = ¾ cup = 6 fluid ounces = 180 mL

16 tablespoons = 1 cup = 8 fluid ounces = 240 mL

INDEX

Note: Page references in *italics* indicate photographs.